MW01130712

Bill Pearl - Images Through the Years

Compiled by Richard R. Thornley Jr, George Coates, Tuesday Coates
Published by Bill Pearl

Copyright © 2015 Bill Pearl

Bill Pearl
P.O. Box 1080
Phoenix, Oregon 97535
Email: support@billpearl.com
Website: www.billpearl.com

ISBN-13 for Soft Cover edition: 978-1-938855-25-2

Cover Image
Photographer - Leo Stern
At Bird Rock, La Jolla, San Diego, CA Circa 1967

NOTICE OF RIGHTS

All rights reserved. No part of this book may be reproduced or transmitted in any form by any means, electronic, mechanical, photocopying, recording, or otherwise, without the prior written permission of the publisher.

FOREWORD

Bill Pearl: A tribute in photographs.

Bill and I have been close friends for almost 60 years. For 20 of those years he ruled the world of national and international bodybuilding, winning all of the top titles against the toughest competition. An extremely modest man, who in spite of his world-wide success, has been endowed with dignity, honesty, and warmth that commands admiration and respect from all.

Bill's friend and colleague Richard 'Rick' Thornley Jr. called my wife Tuesday and I to ask if we would assist him in compiling a tribute to Bill using photographs. We jumped at the chance.

What follows are images of Bill from 1951 to 1971, some of which have never been published. Let the images speak for themselves.

Enjoy!

George Coates
San Diego, California

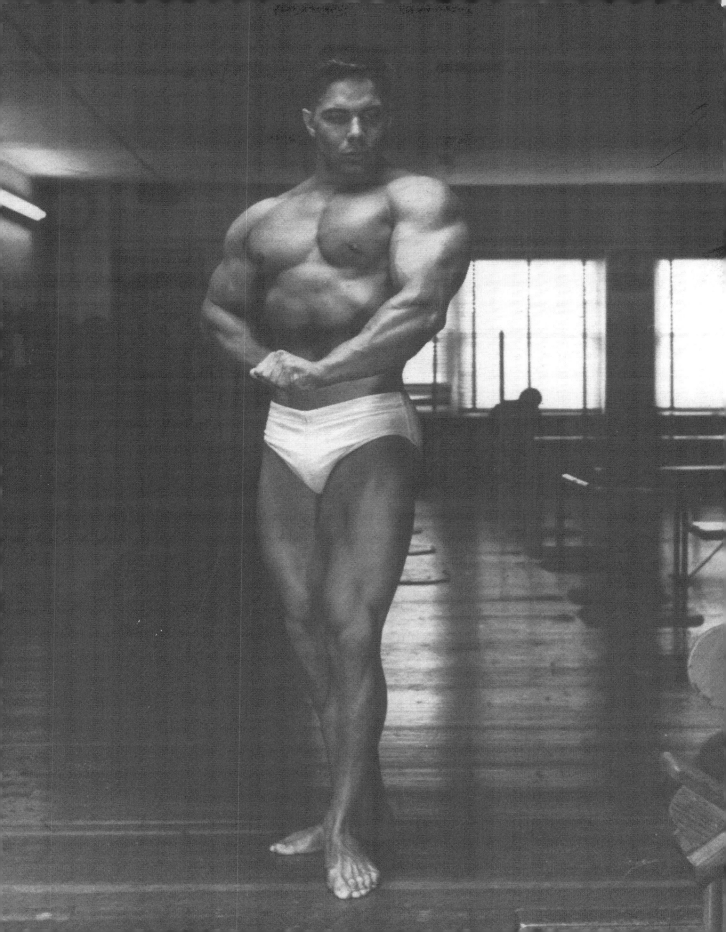

Image Number One
Photographer - Leo Stern
At Stern's Gym, San Diego, CA
Circa 1953 thru 1961

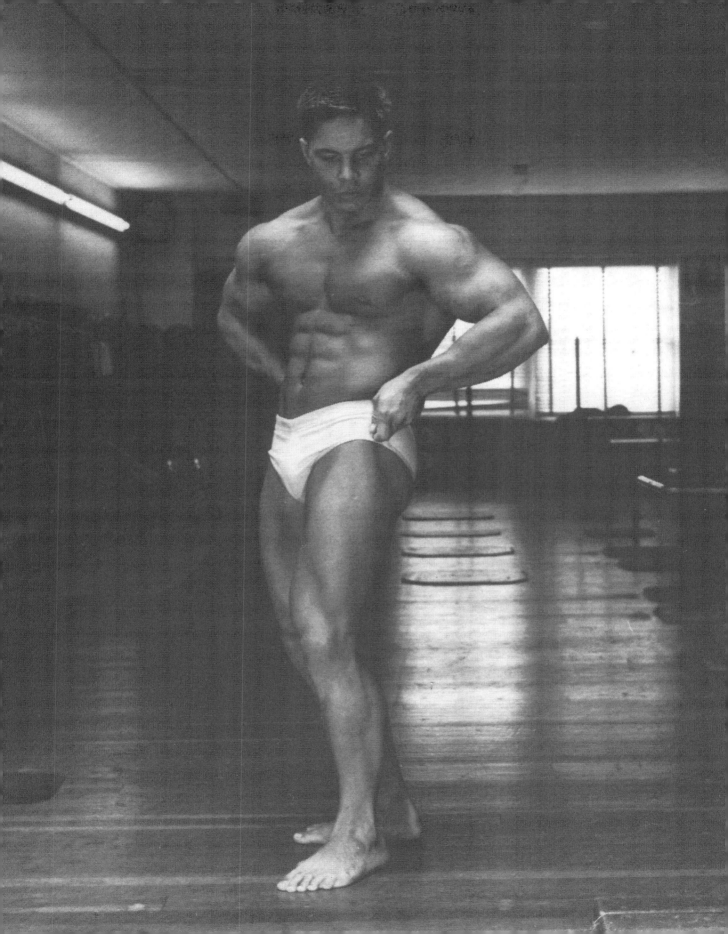

Image Number Two
Photographer - Leo Stern
At Stern's Gym, San Diego, CA
Circa 1953 thru 1961

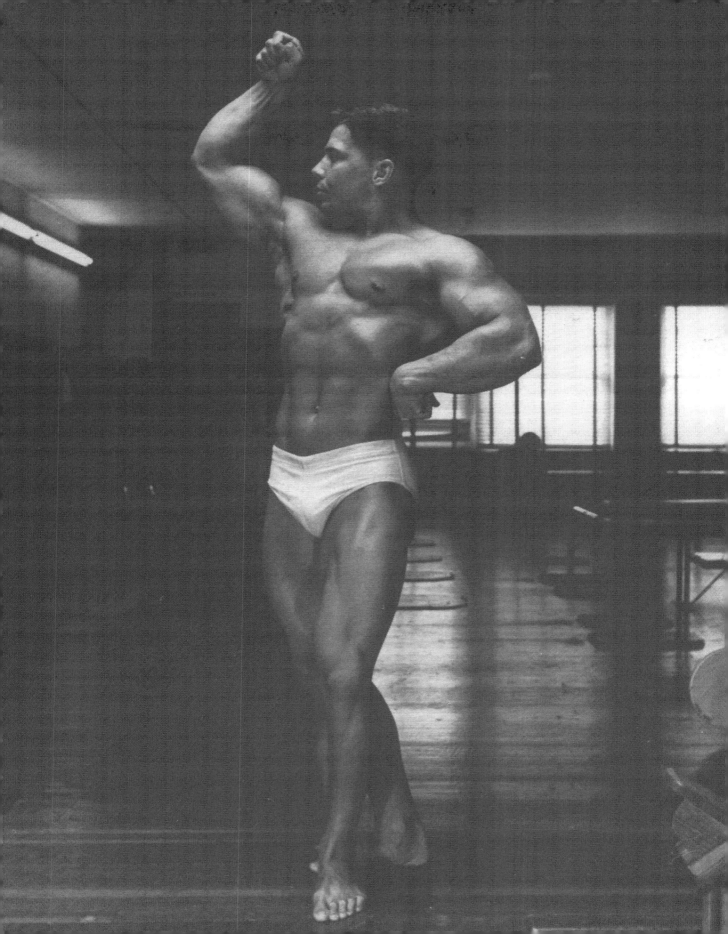

Image Number Three
Photographer - Leo Stern
At Stern's Gym, San Diego, CA
Circa 1953 thru 1961

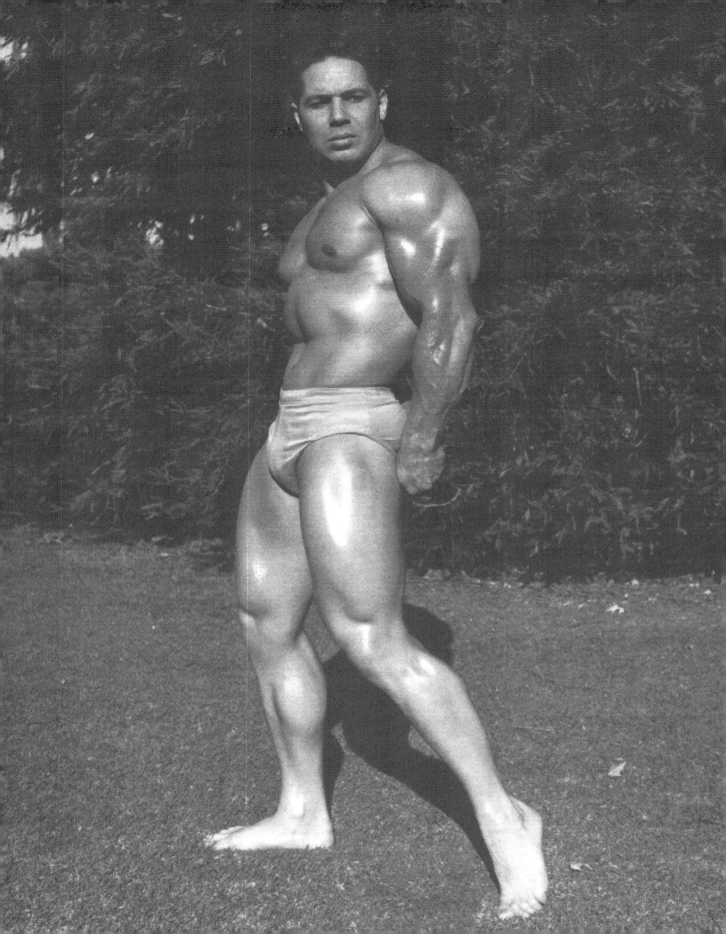

Image Number Four
Photographer - Leo Stern
At Balboa Park, San Diego, CA
Circa 1960

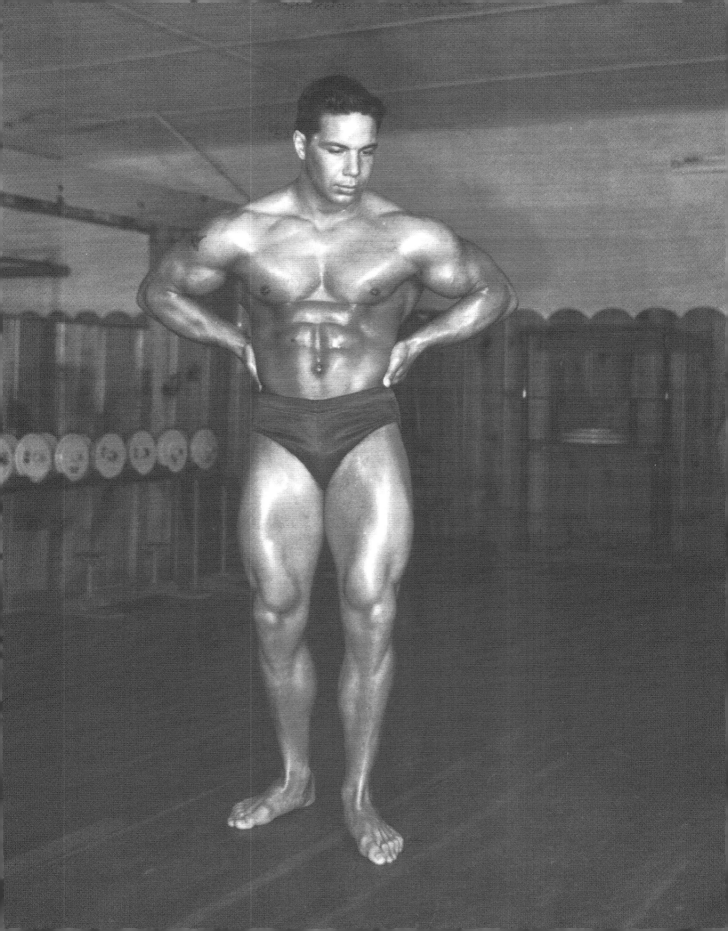

Image Number Five
Photographer - Leo Stern
At Stern's Gym, San Diego, CA
Circa 1953 thru 1961

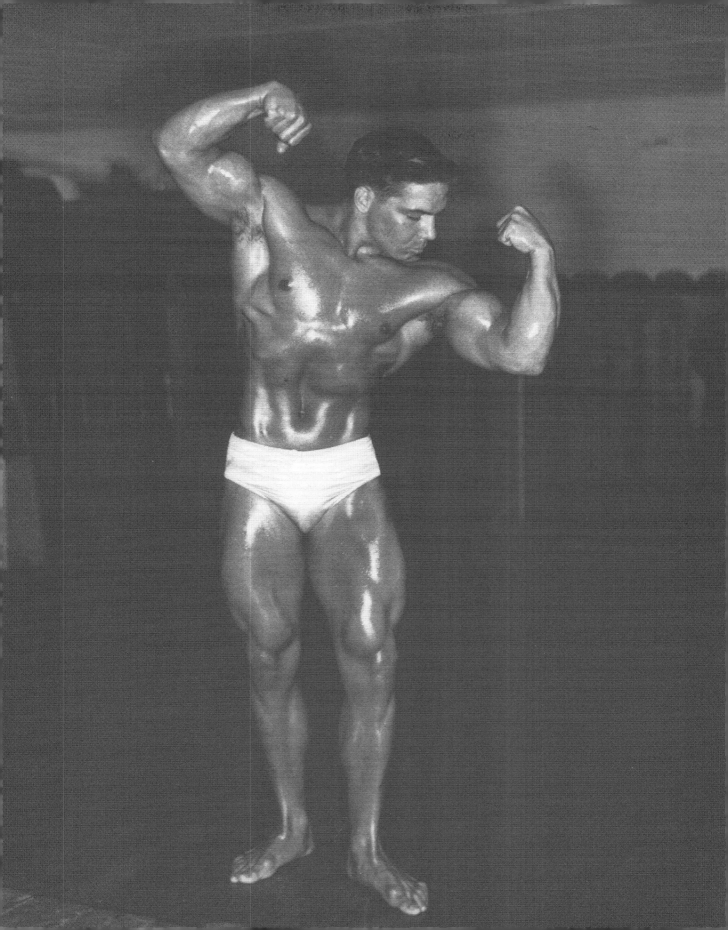

Image Number Six
Photographer - Leo Stern
At Stern's Gym, San Diego, CA
Circa 1953 thru 1961

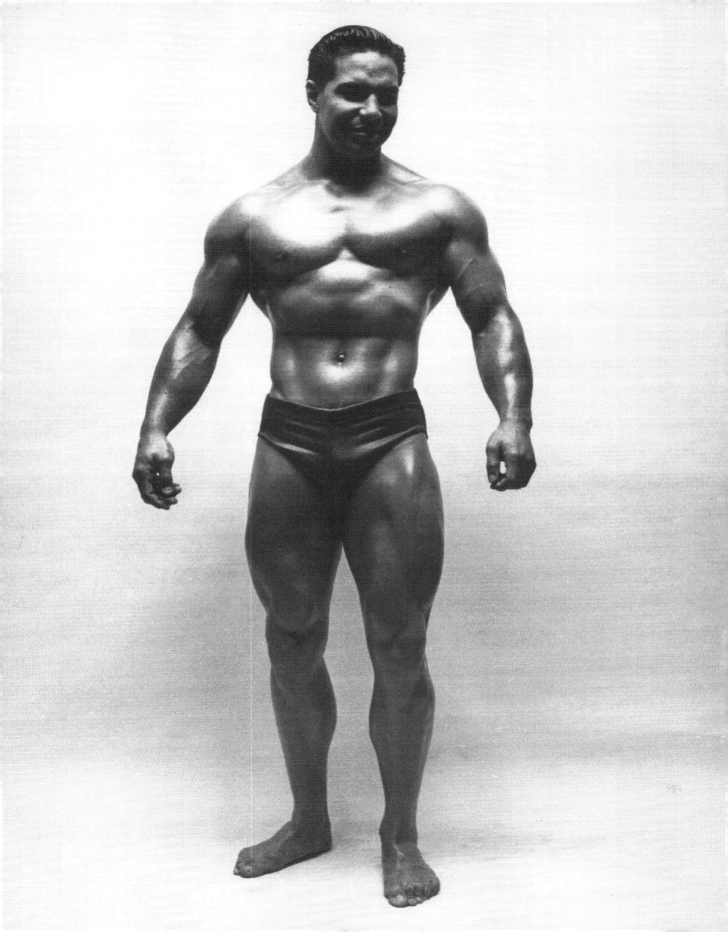

Image Number Seven
Photographer - Leo Stern
At Stern's Gym, San Diego, CA
Circa 1953 thru 1961

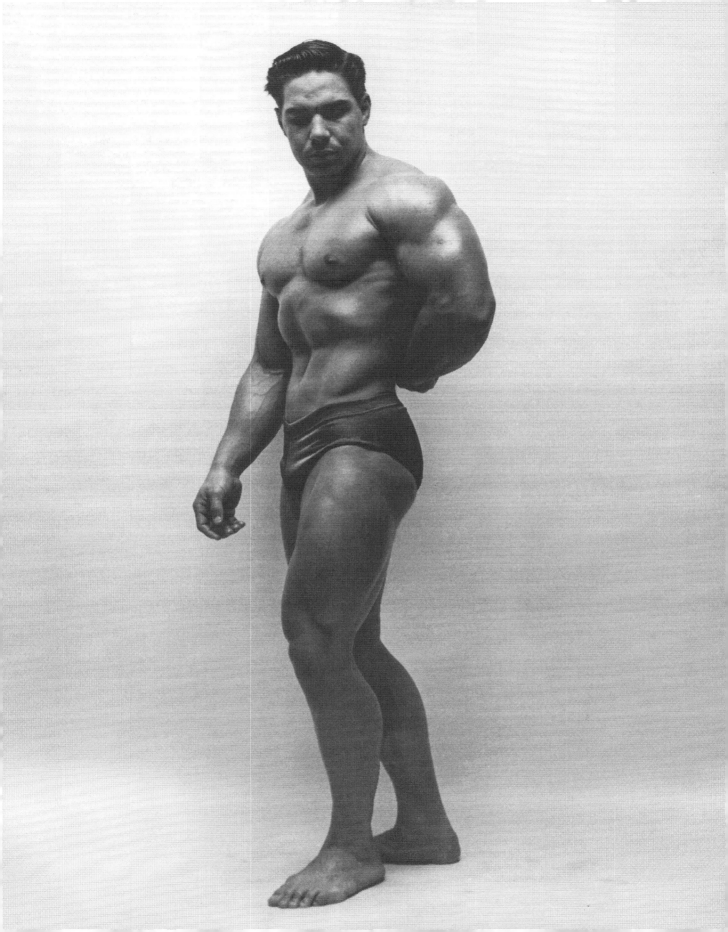

Image Number Eight
Photographer - Leo Stern
At Stern's Gym, San Diego, CA
Circa 1953 thru 1961

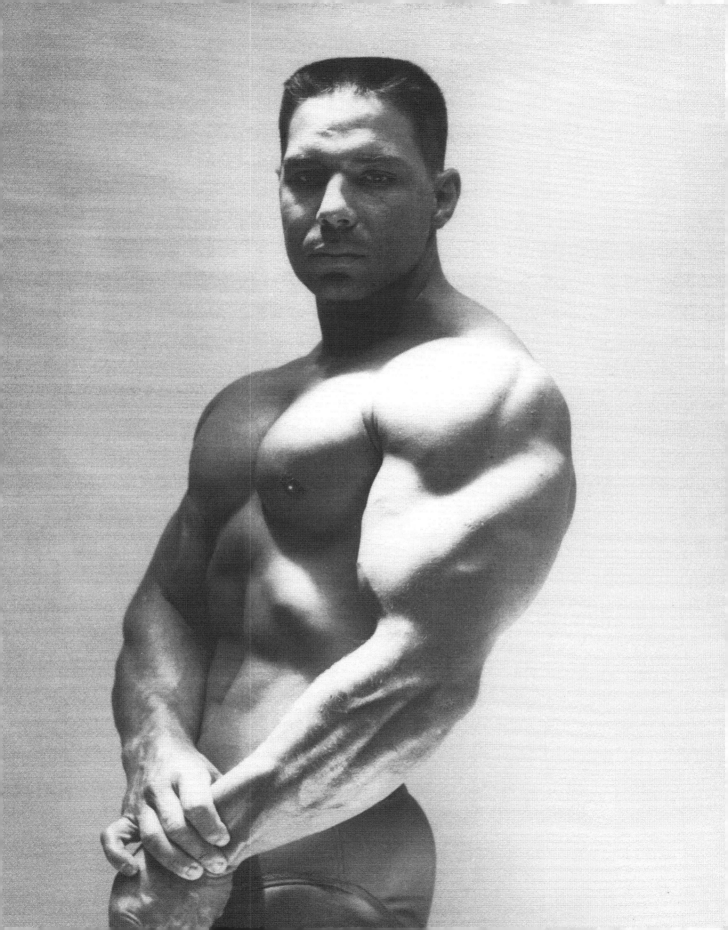

Image Number Nine
Photographer - Leo Stern
At Stern's Gym, San Diego, CA
Circa 1953 thru 1961

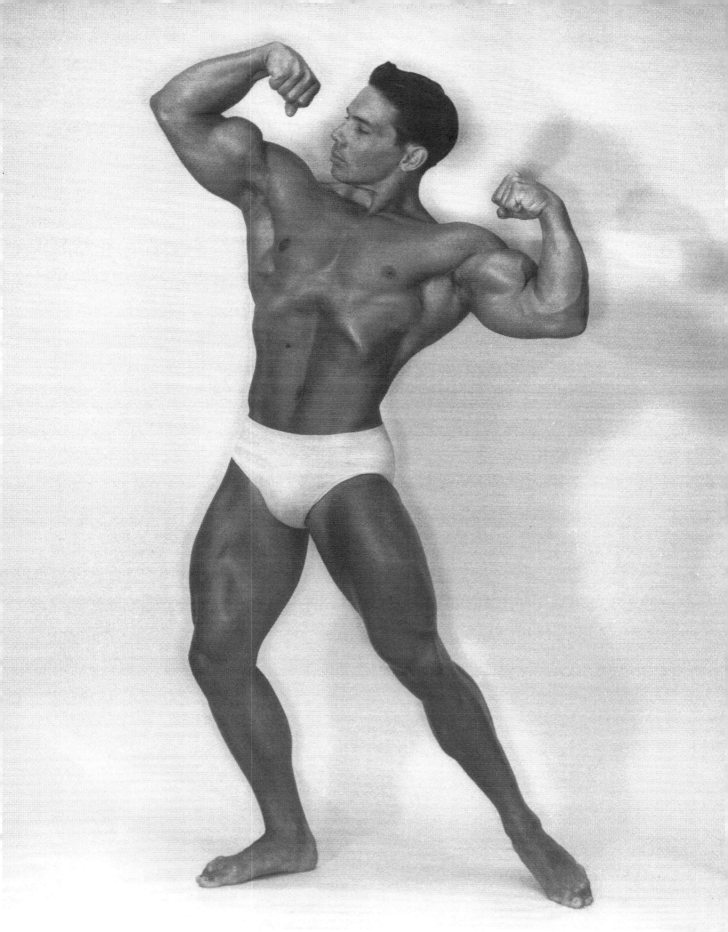

Image Number Ten
Photographer - Leo Stern
At Stern's Gym, San Diego, CA
Circa 1953 thru 1961

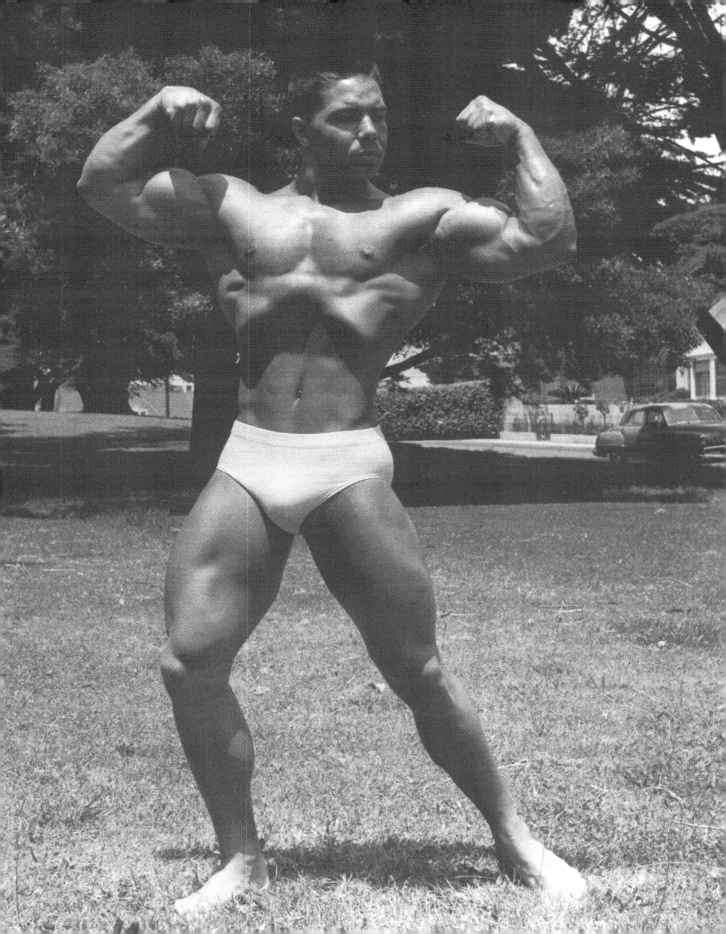

Image Number Eleven
Photographer - Leo Stern
At Balboa Park, San Diego, CA
Circa 1960

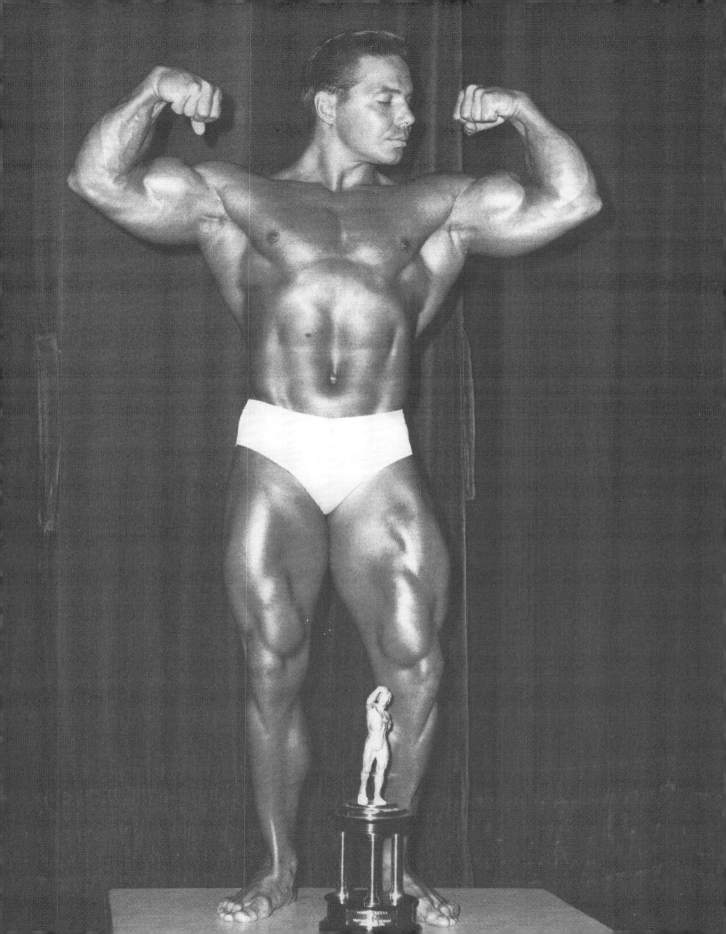

Image Number Twelve
Photographer – Paul Hawker
At the 1961 NABBA Mr Universe Contest at the
Victoria Palace Theatre, London England

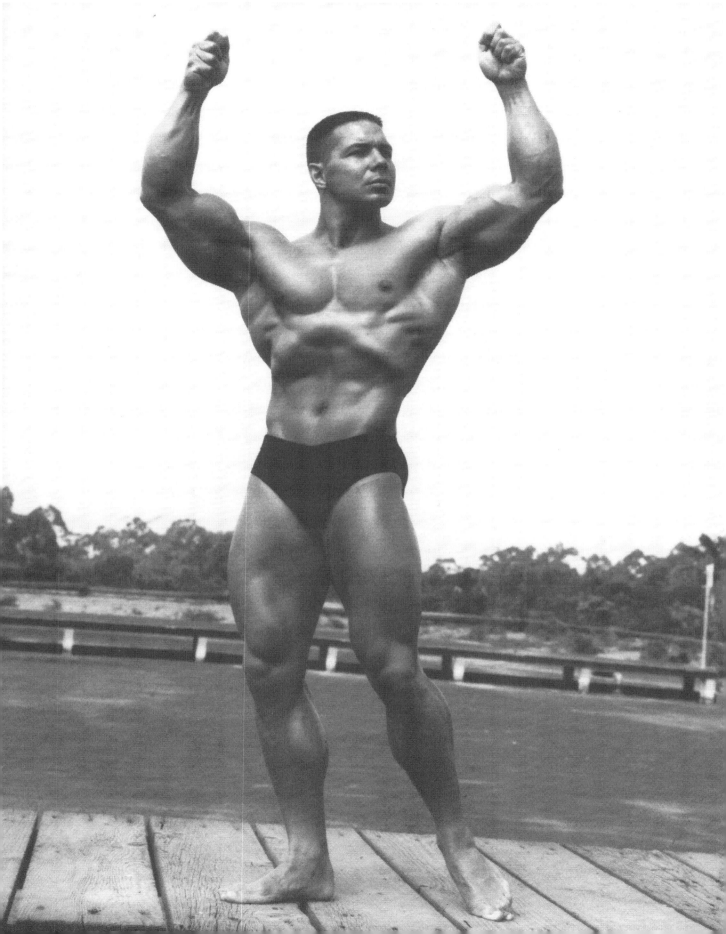

Image Number Thirteen
Photographer - Leo Stern
At the casting pool in North Park area of San Diego, CA
Circa 1962 thru 1965

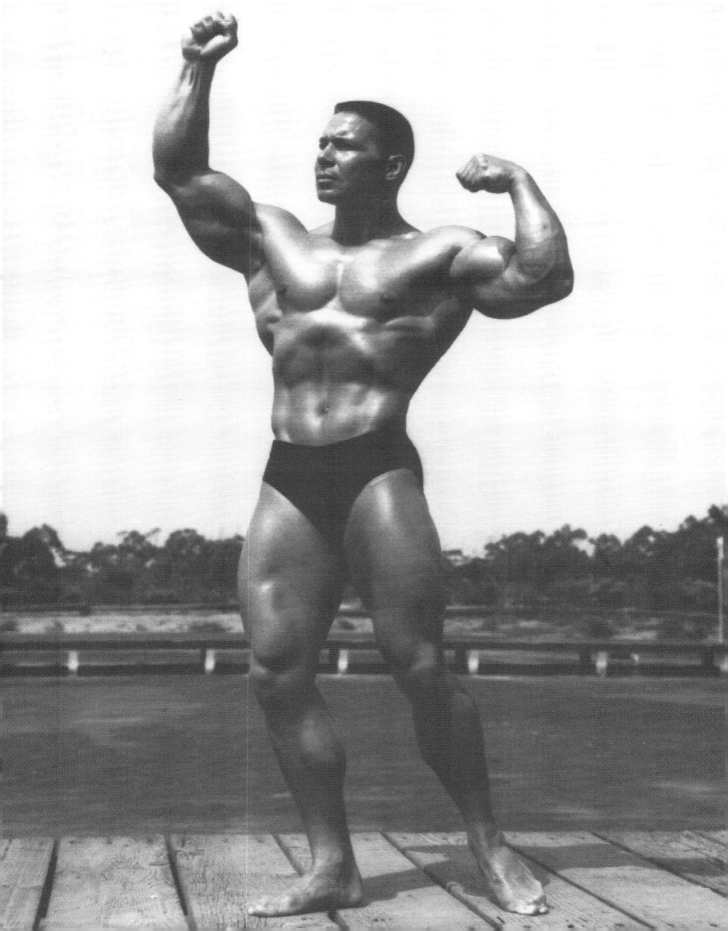

Image Number Fourteen
Photographer - Leo Stern
At the casting pool in North Park area of San Diego, CA
Circa 1962 thru 1965

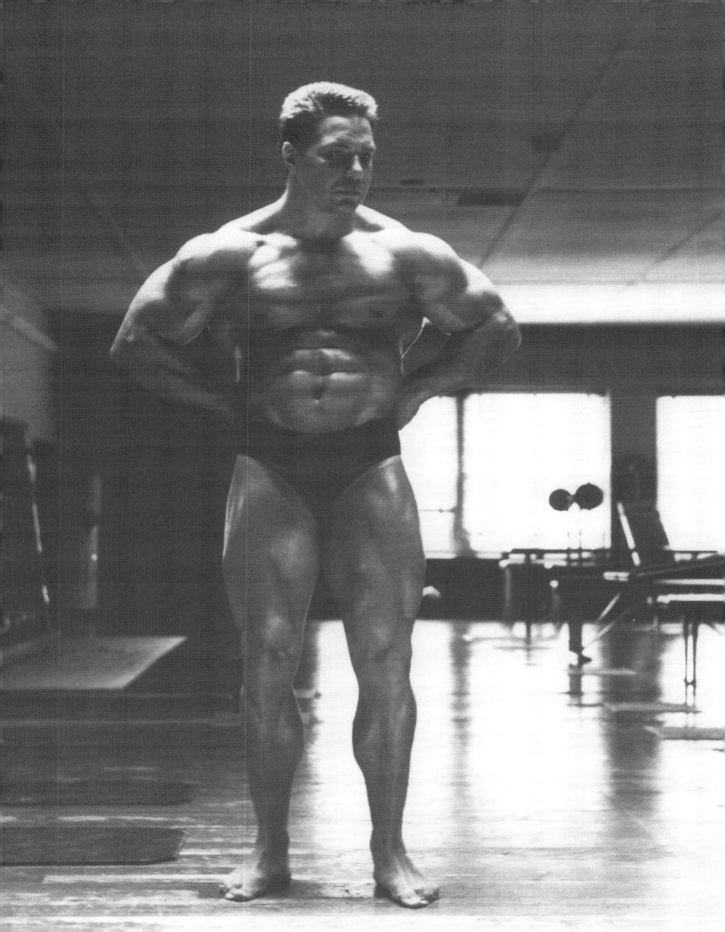

Image Number Fifteen
Photographer - Leo Stern
At Stern's Gym, San Diego, CA
Circa 1963 thru 1966

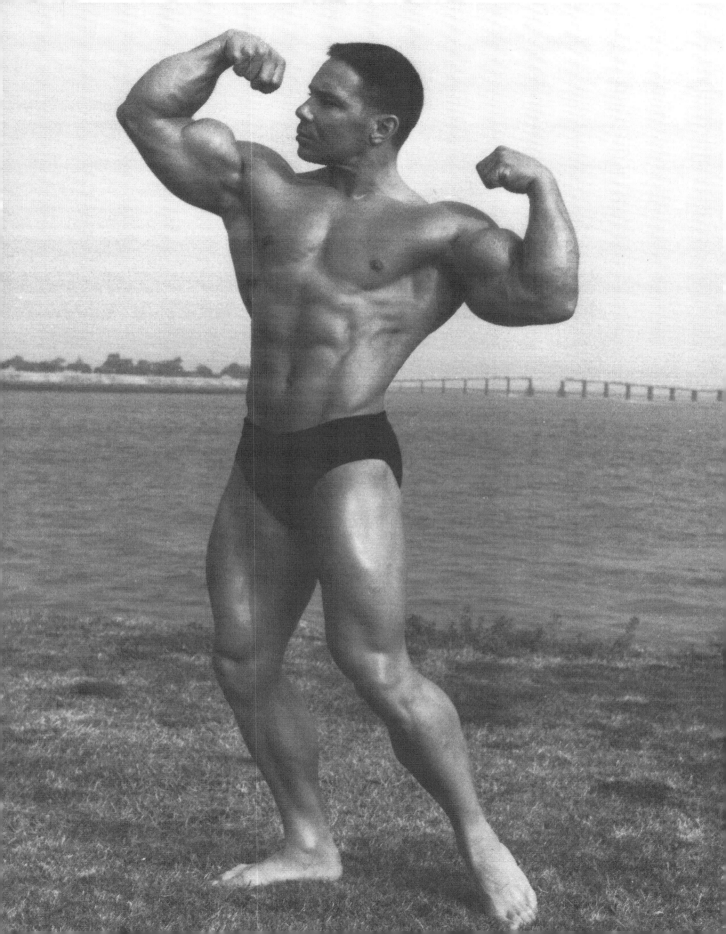

Image Number Sixteen
Photographer - Leo Stern
At Mission Bay, San Diego, CA
Circa 1963 thru 1966

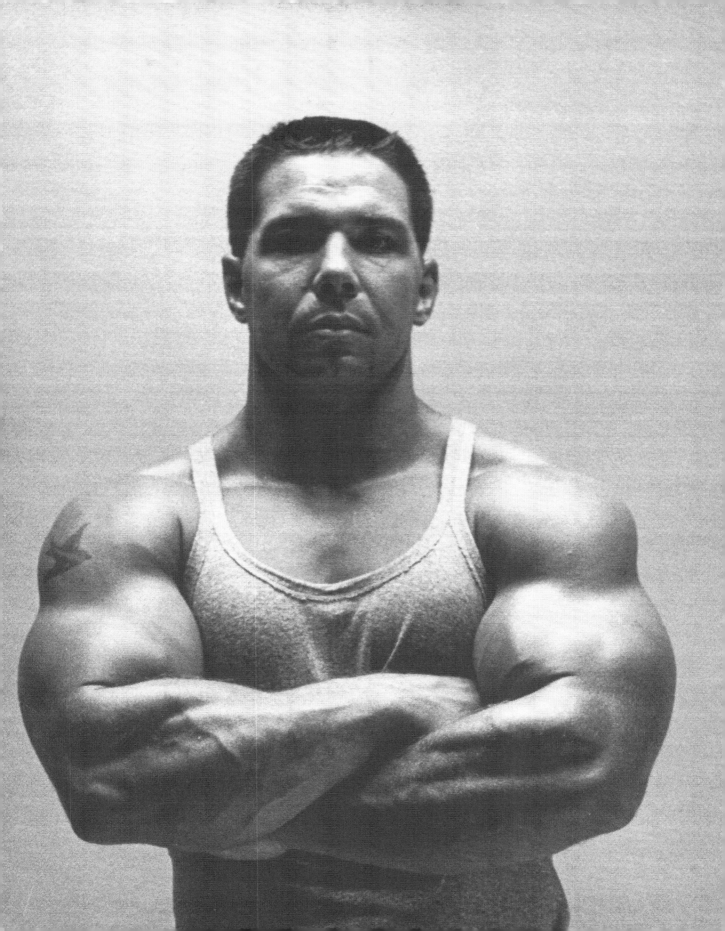

Image Number Seventeen
Photographer - Leo Stern
At Stern's Gym, San Diego, CA
Circa 1963 thru 1966

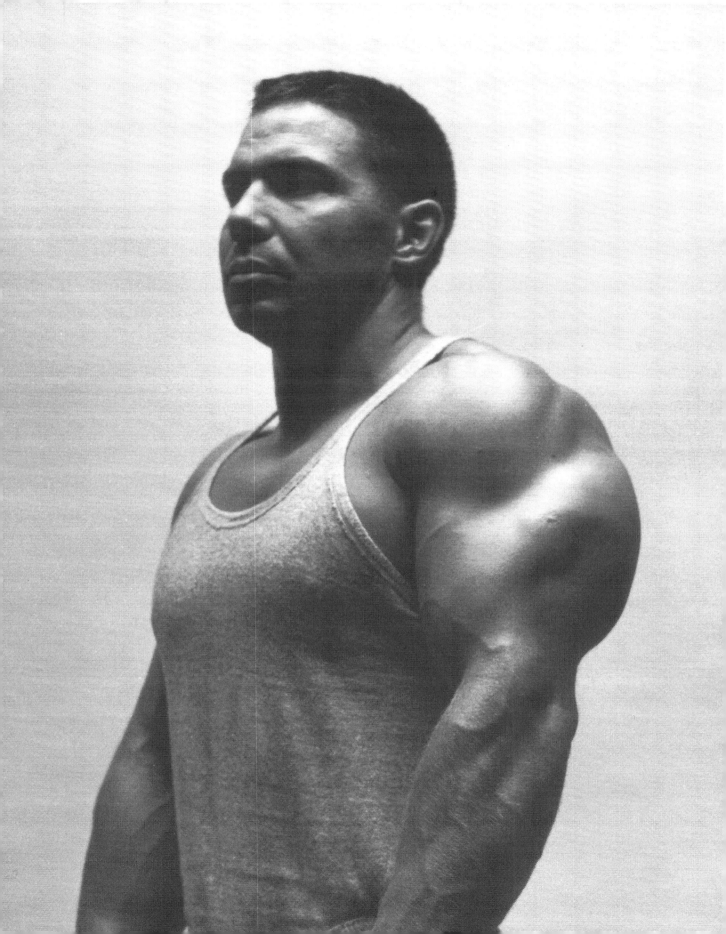

Image Number Eighteen
Photographer - Leo Stern
At Stern's Gym, San Diego, CA
Circa 1963 thru 1966

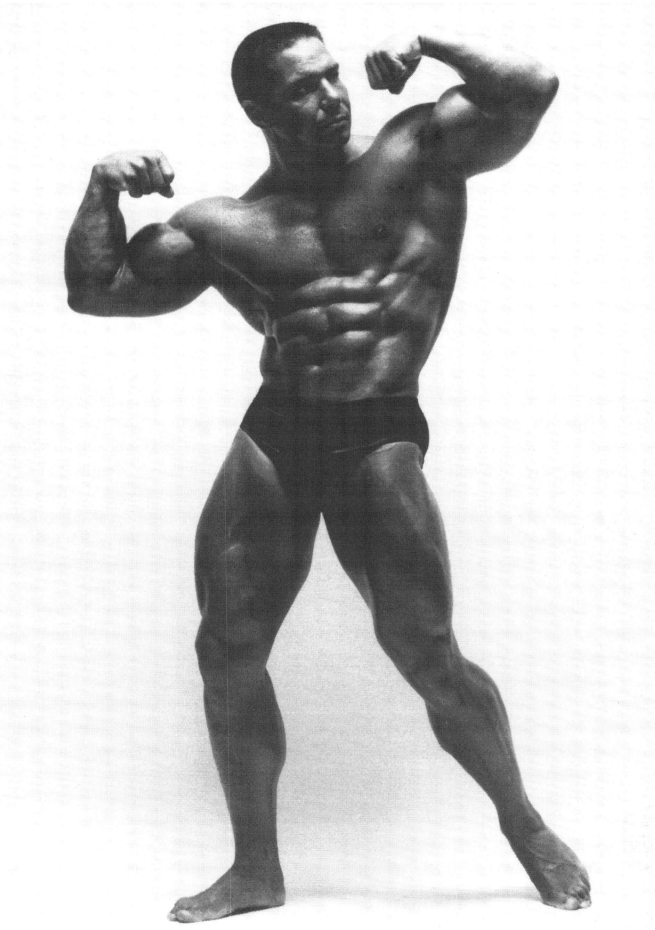

Image Number Nineteen
Photographer - Leo Stern
At Stern's Gym, San Diego, CA
Circa 1963 thru 1966

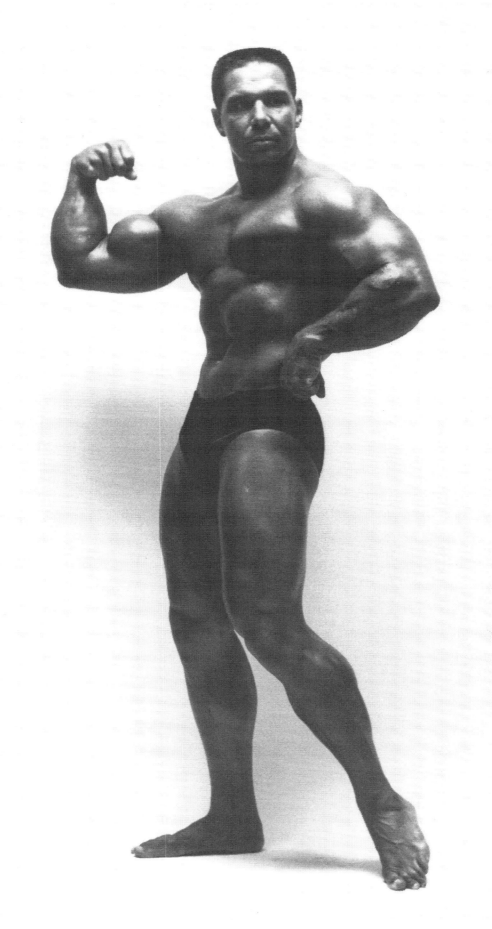

Image Number Twenty
Photographer - Leo Stern
At Stern's Gym, San Diego, CA
Circa 1963 thru 1966

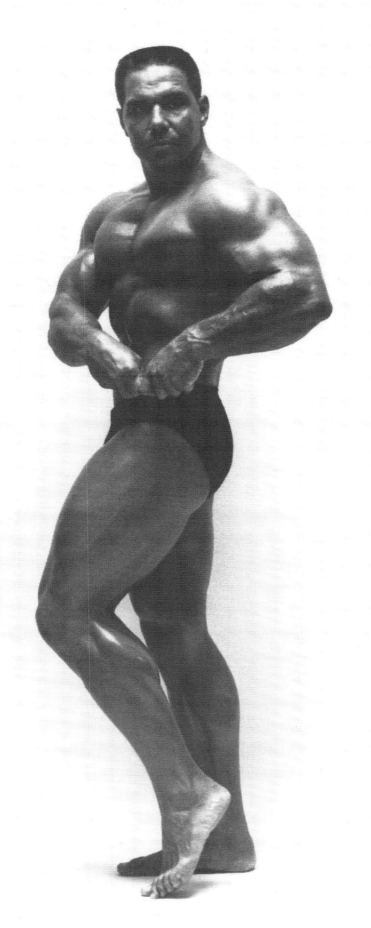

Image Number Twenty-One
Photographer - Leo Stern
At Stern's Gym, San Diego, CA
Circa 1963 thru 1966

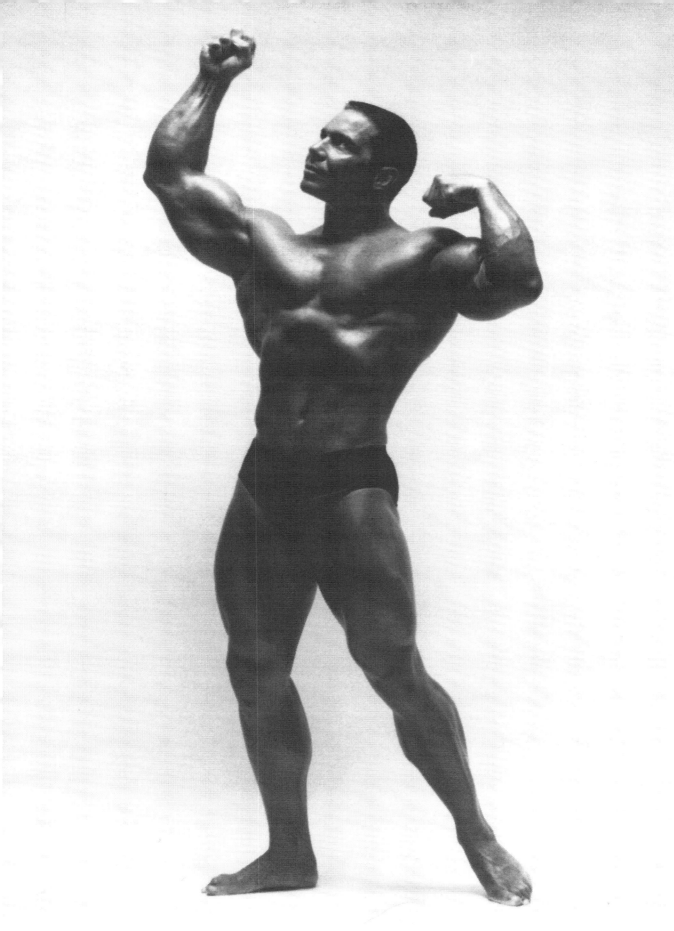

Image Number Twenty-Two
Photographer - Leo Stern
At Stern's Gym, San Diego, CA
Circa 1963 thru 1966

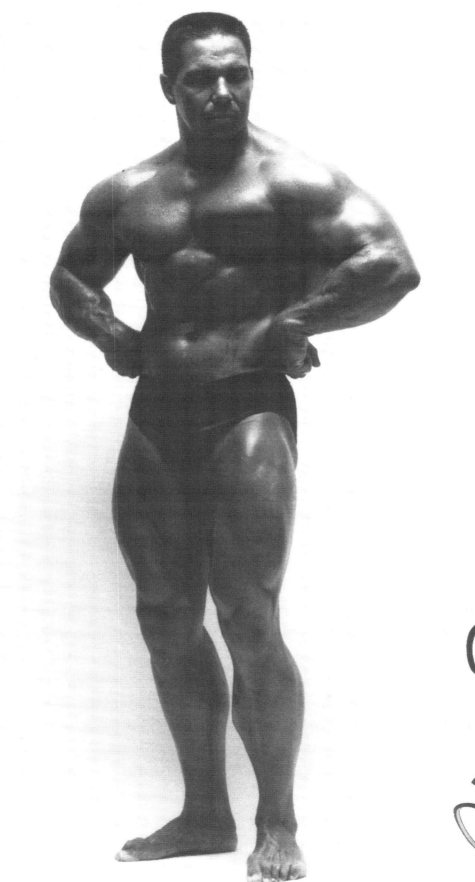

Bill Pearl

Image Number Twenty-Three
Photographer - Leo Stern
At Stern's Gym, San Diego, CA
Circa 1963 thru 1966

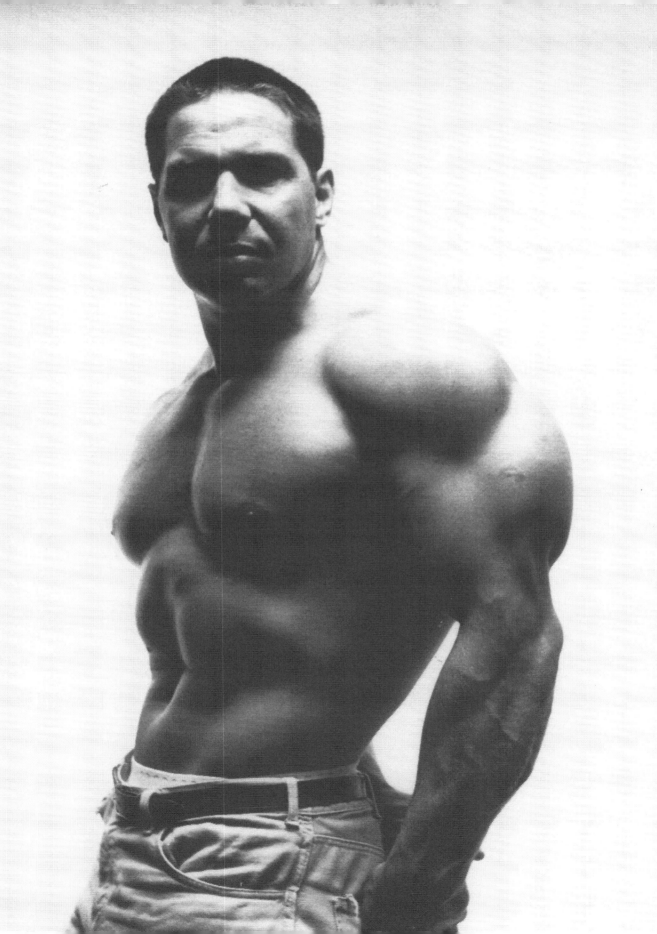

Image Number Twenty-Four
Photographer - Leo Stern
At Stern's Gym, San Diego, CA
Circa 1963 thru 1966

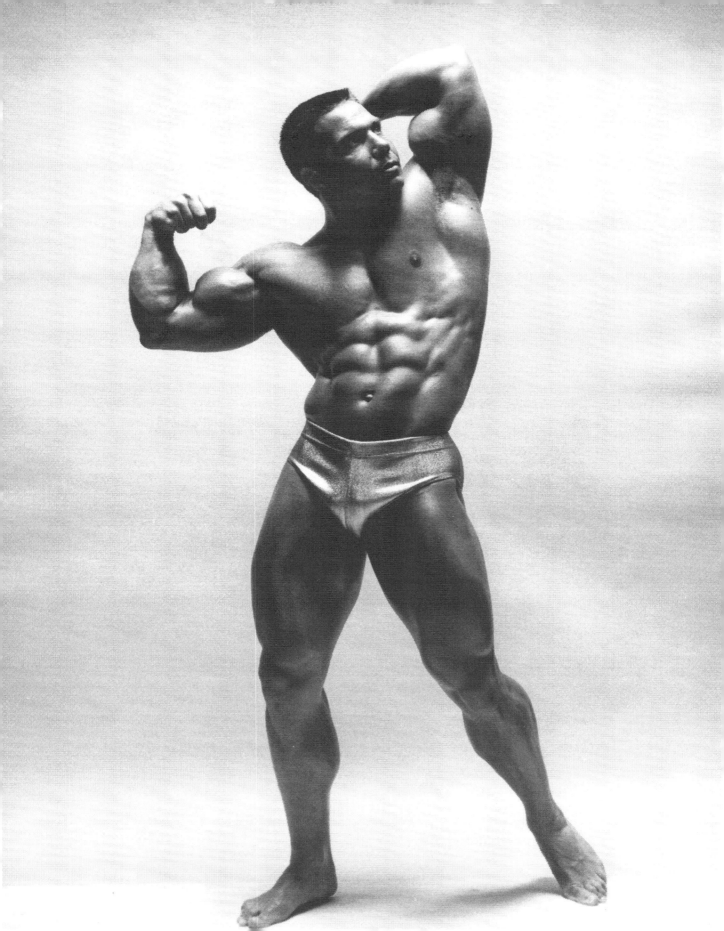

Image Number Twenty-Five
Photographer - Leo Stern
At Stern's Gym, San Diego, CA
Circa 1966 thru 1968

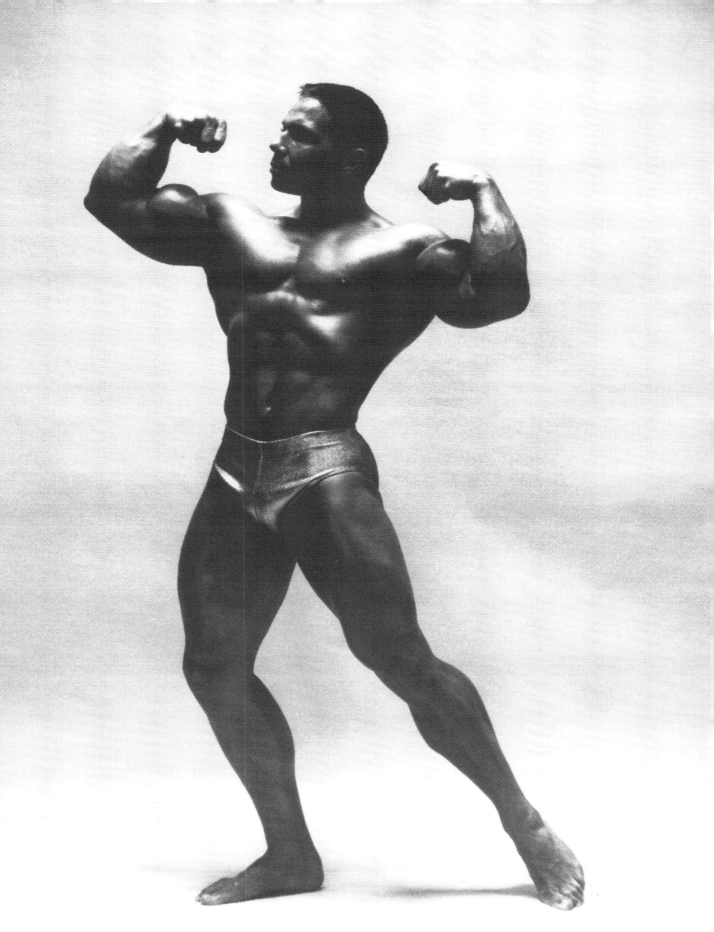

Image Number Twenty-Six
Photographer - Leo Stern
At Stern's Gym, San Diego, CA
Circa 1966 thru 1968

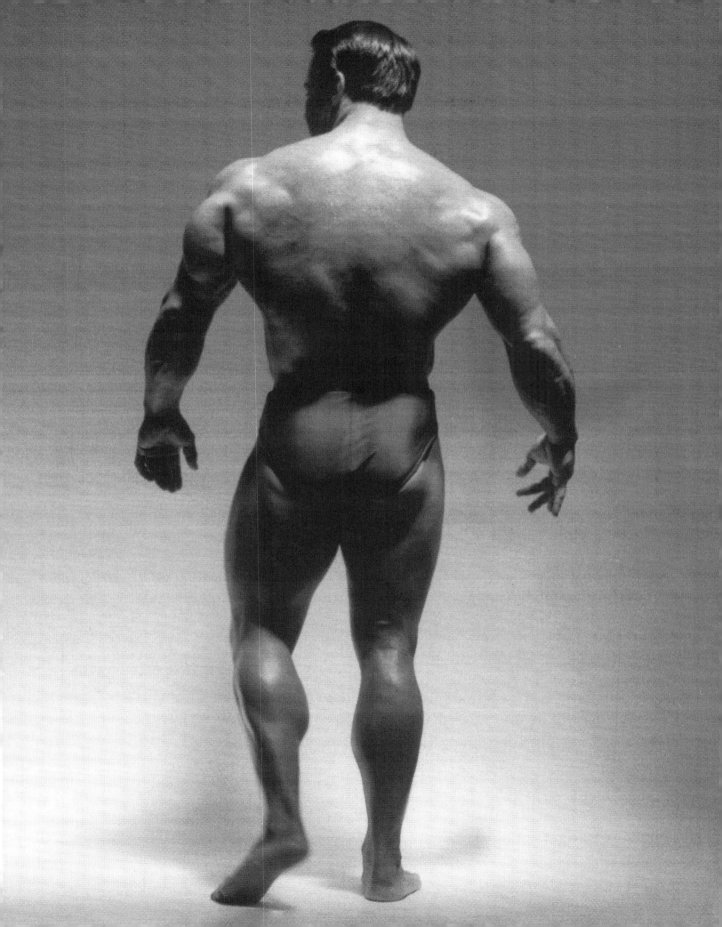

Image Number Twenty-Seven
Photographer - Leo Stern
At Stern's Gym, San Diego, CA
Circa 1966 thru 1968

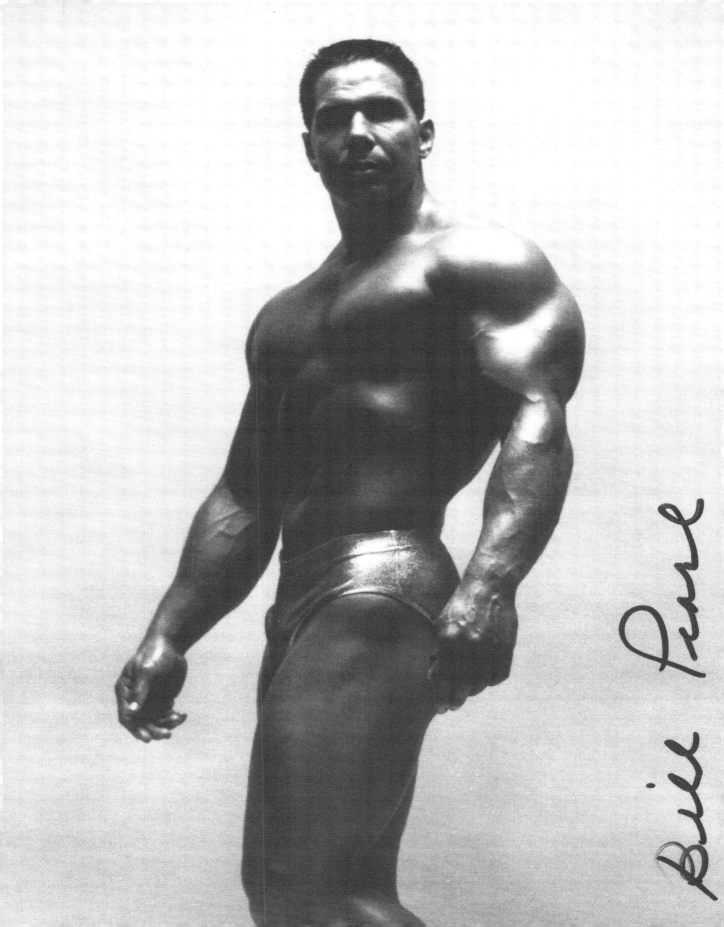

Image Number Twenty-Eight
Photographer - Leo Stern
At Stern's Gym, San Diego, CA
Circa 1966 thru 1968

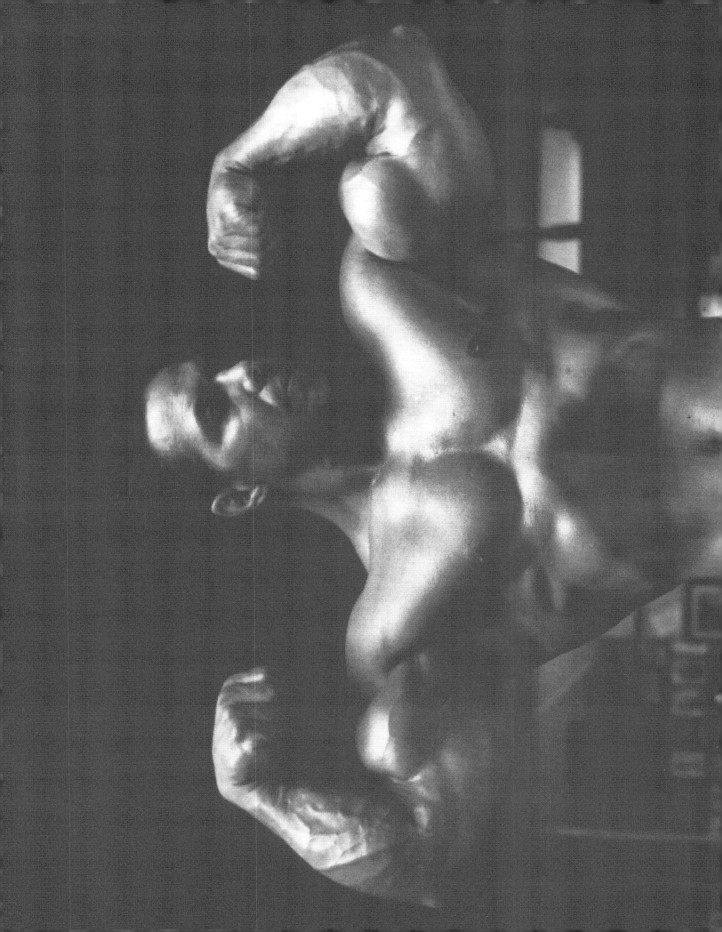

Image Number Twenty-Nine
Photographer - Leo Stern
At Stern's Gym, San Diego, CA
Circa 1966 thru 1968

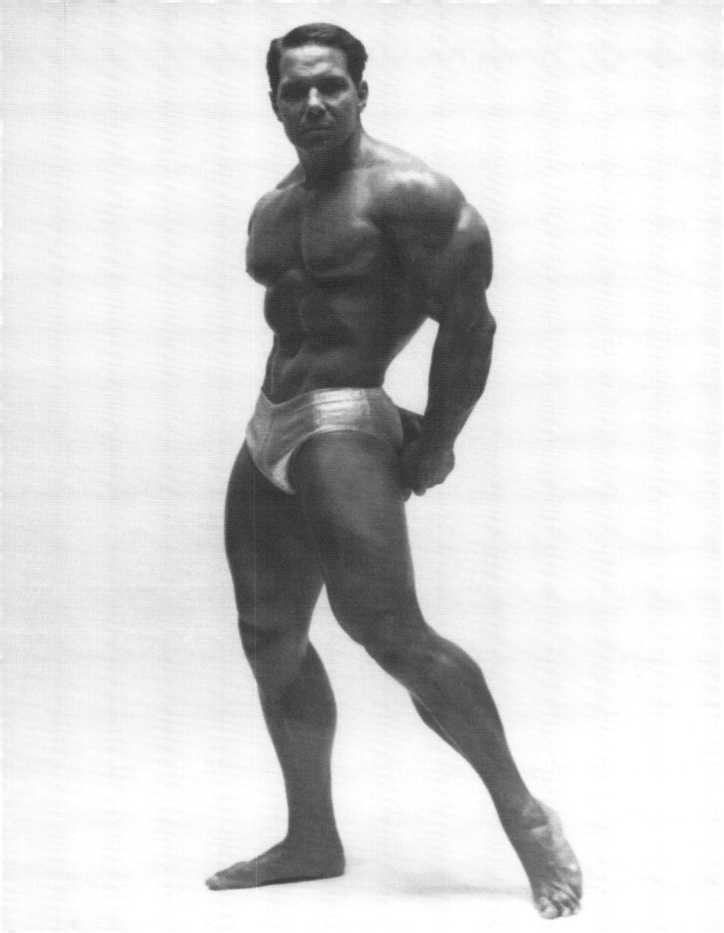

Image Number Thirty
Photographer - Leo Stern
At Stern's Gym, San Diego, CA
Circa 1966 thru 1968

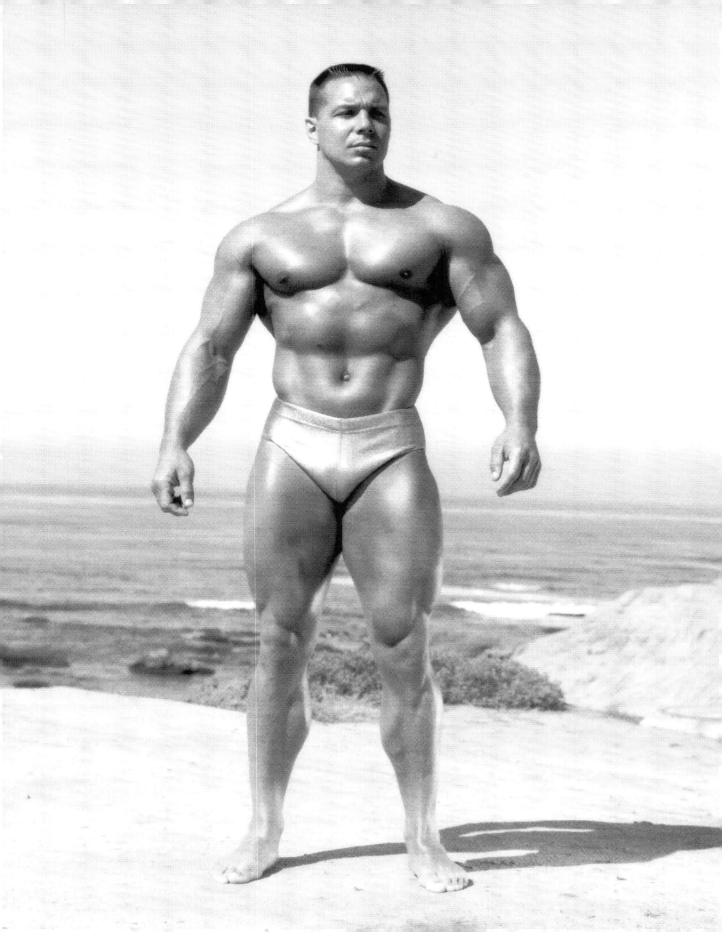

Image Number Thirty-One
Photographer - Leo Stern
At Bird Rock, La Jolla, San Diego, CA
Circa 1967

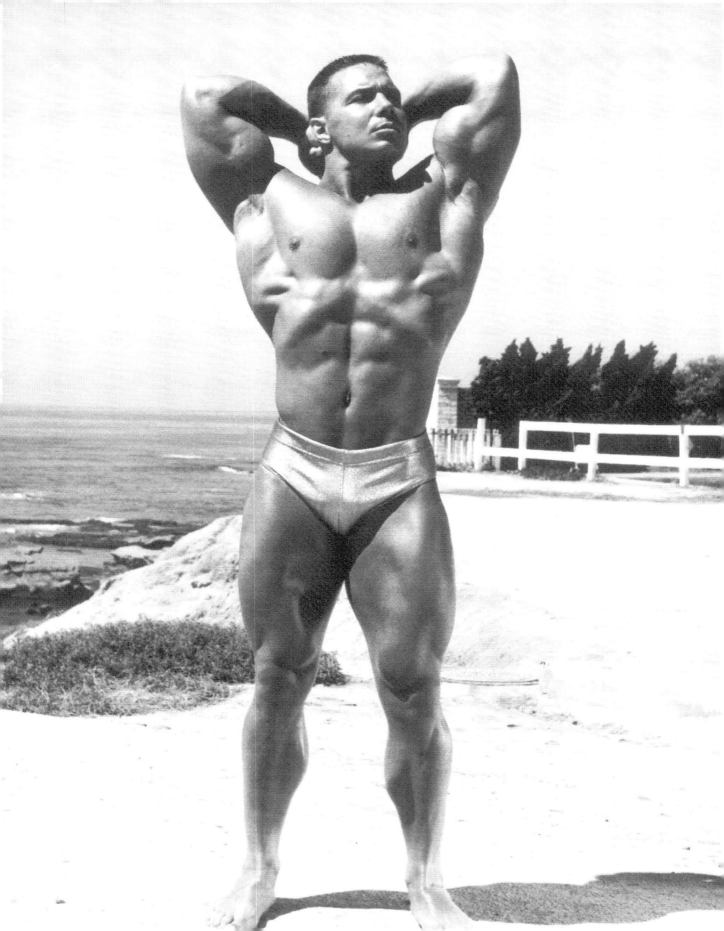

Image Number Thirty-Two
Photographer - Leo Stern
At Bird Rock, La Jolla, San Diego, CA
Circa 1967

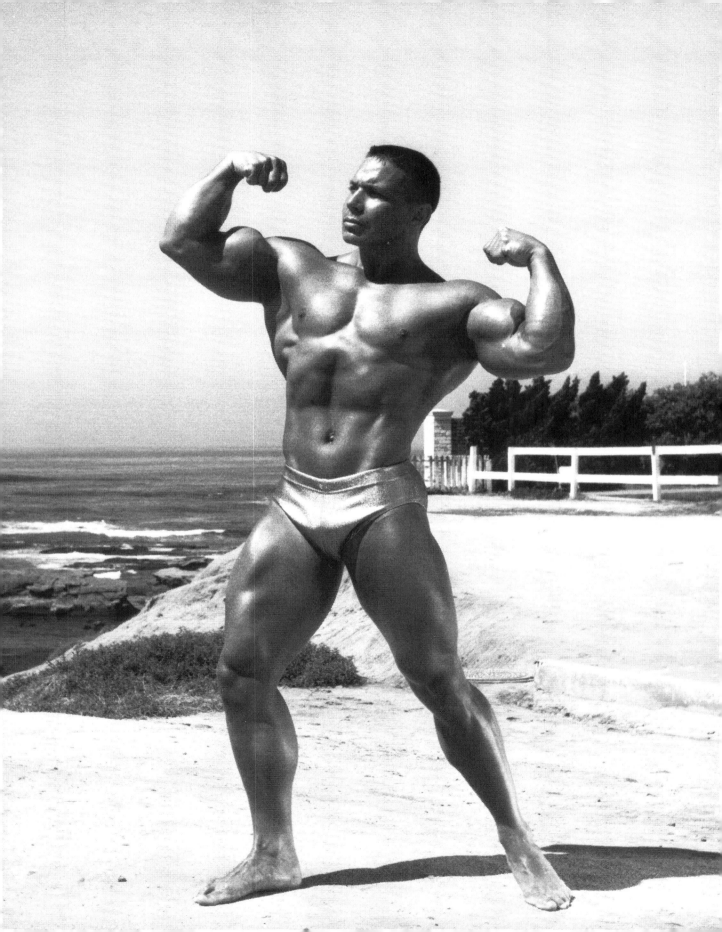

Image Number Thirty-Three
Photographer - Leo Stern
At Bird Rock, La Jolla, San Diego, CA
Circa 1967

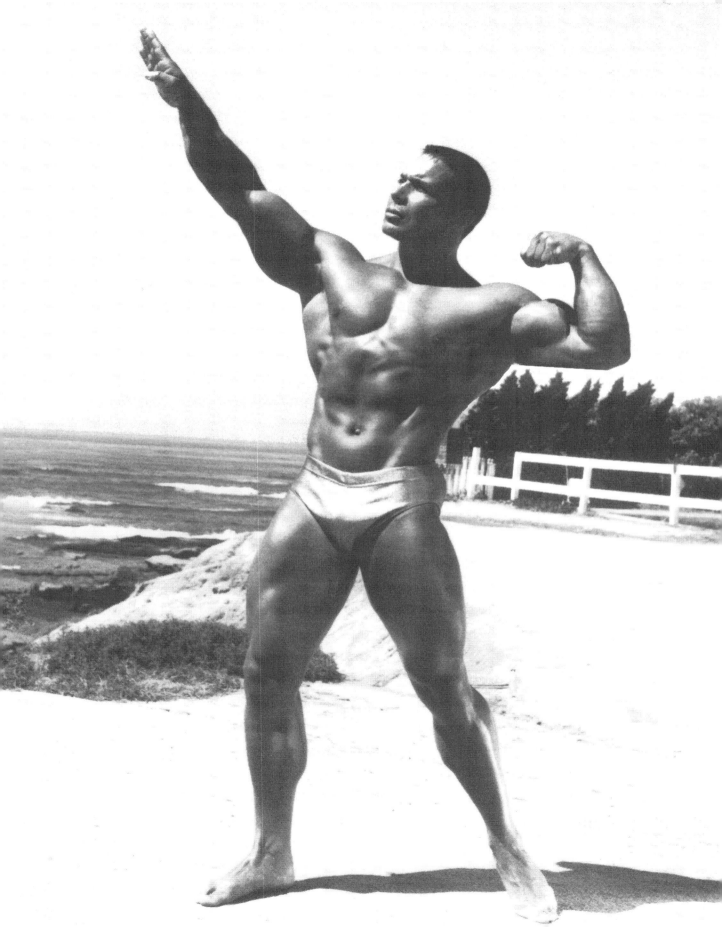

Image Number Thirty-Four
Photographer - Leo Stern
At Bird Rock, La Jolla, San Diego, CA
Circa 1967

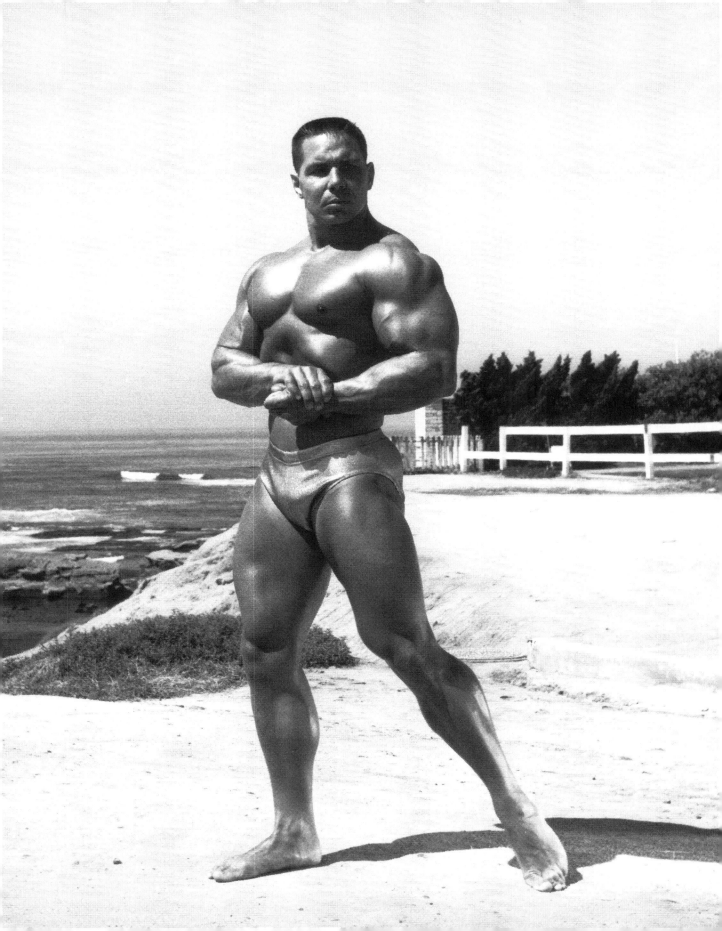

Image Number Thirty-Five
Photographer - Leo Stern
At Bird Rock, La Jolla, San Diego, CA
Circa 1967

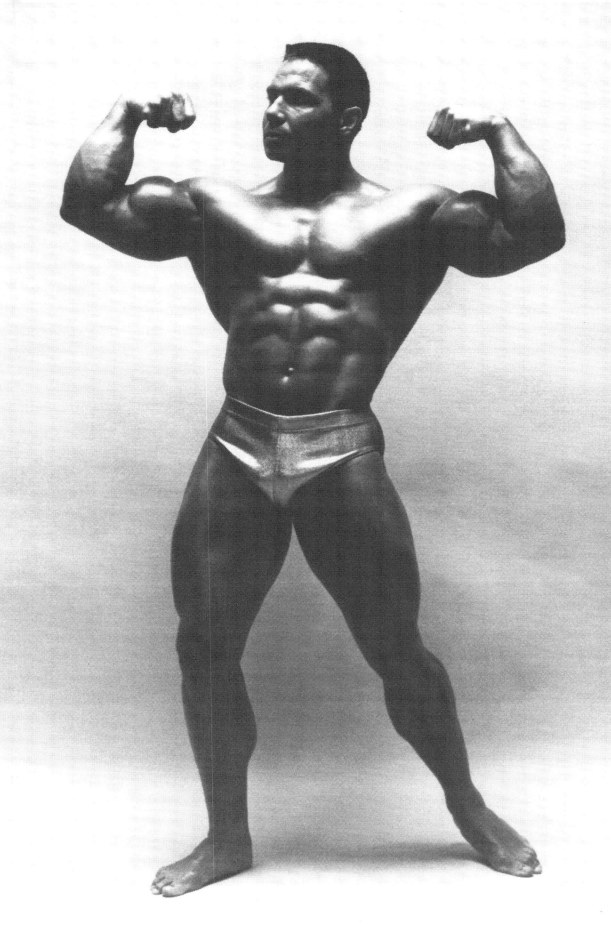

Image Number Thirty-Six
Photographer - Leo Stern
At Stern's Gym, San Diego, CA
Circa 1966 thru 1968

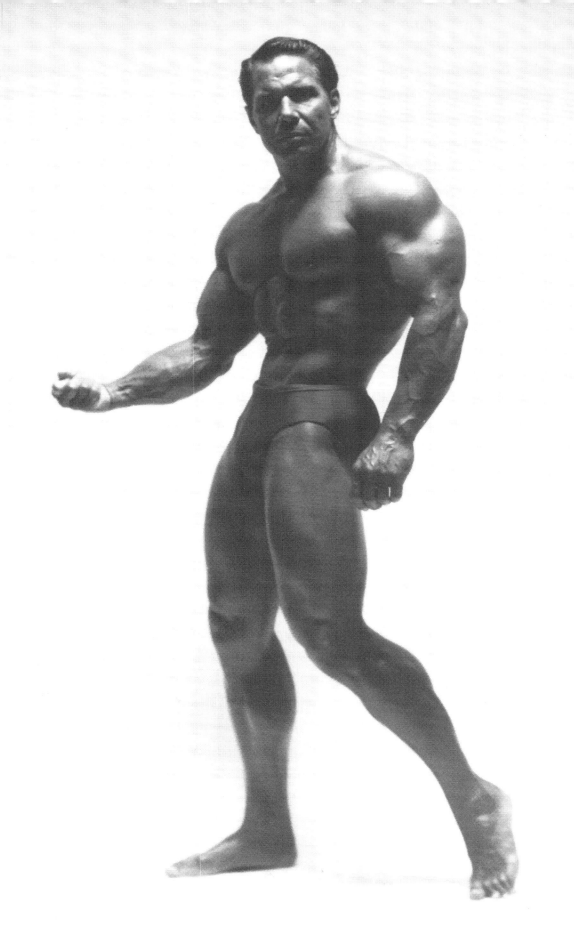

Image Number Thirty-Seven
Photographer - Leo Stern
At Stern's Gym, San Diego, CA
Circa 1970 thru 1971

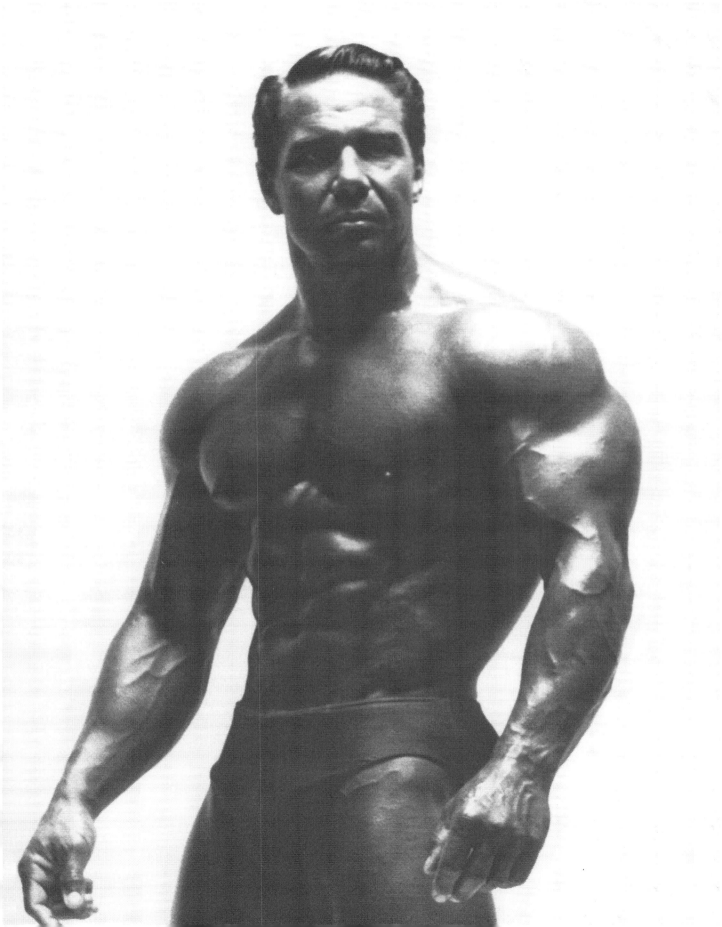

Image Number Thirty-Eight
Photographer - Leo Stern
At Stern's Gym, San Diego, CA
Circa 1970 thru 1971

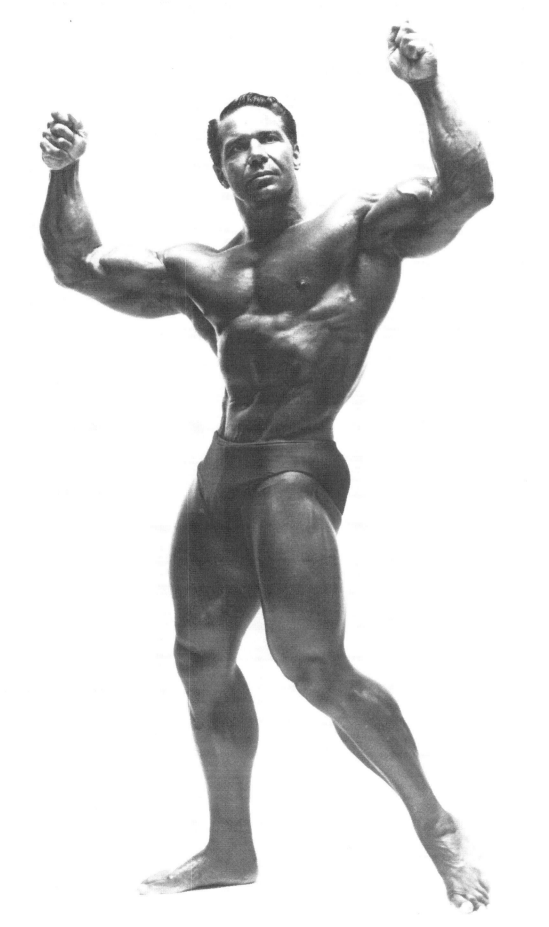

Image Number Thirty-Nine
Photographer - Leo Stern
At Stern's Gym, San Diego, CA
Circa 1970 thru 1971

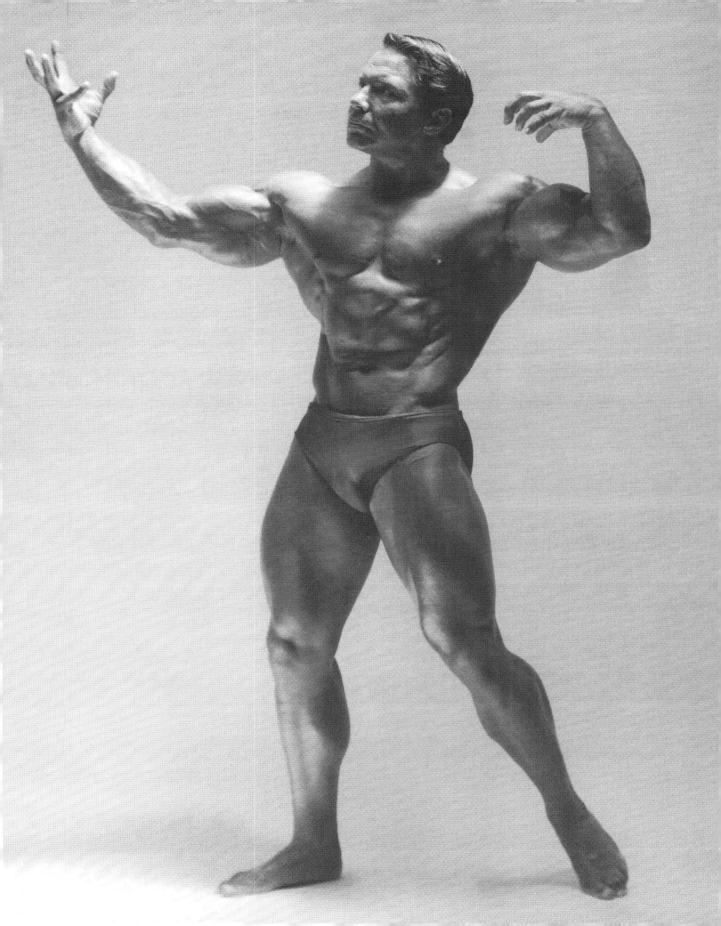

Image Number Forty
Photographer - Leo Stern
At Stern's Gym, San Diego, CA
Circa 1970 thru 1971

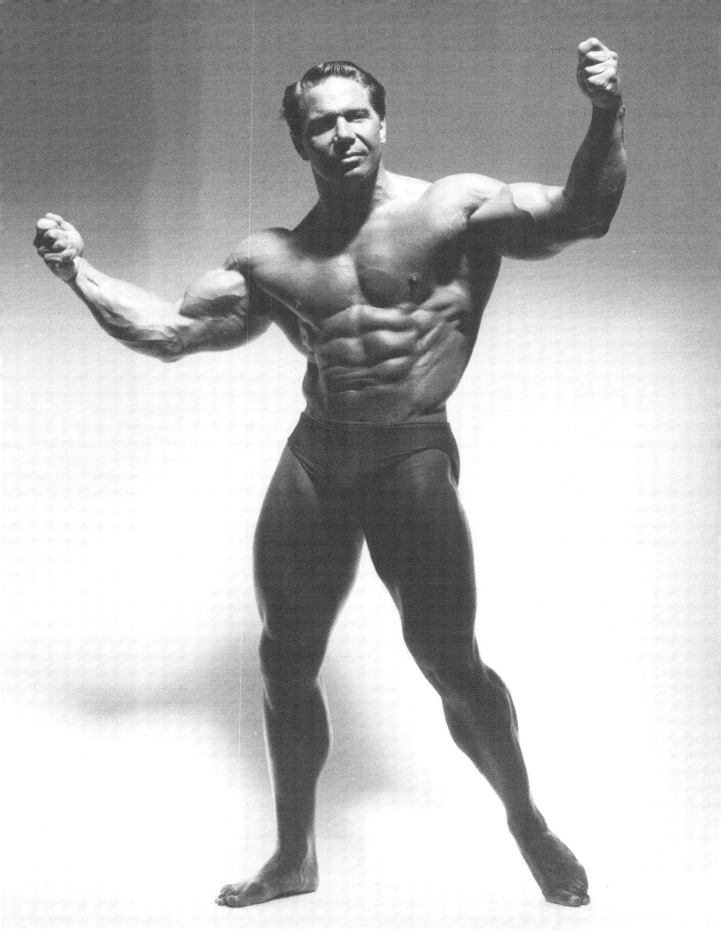

Image Number Forty-One
Photographer - Leo Stern
At Stern's Gym, San Diego, CA
Circa 1970 thru 1971

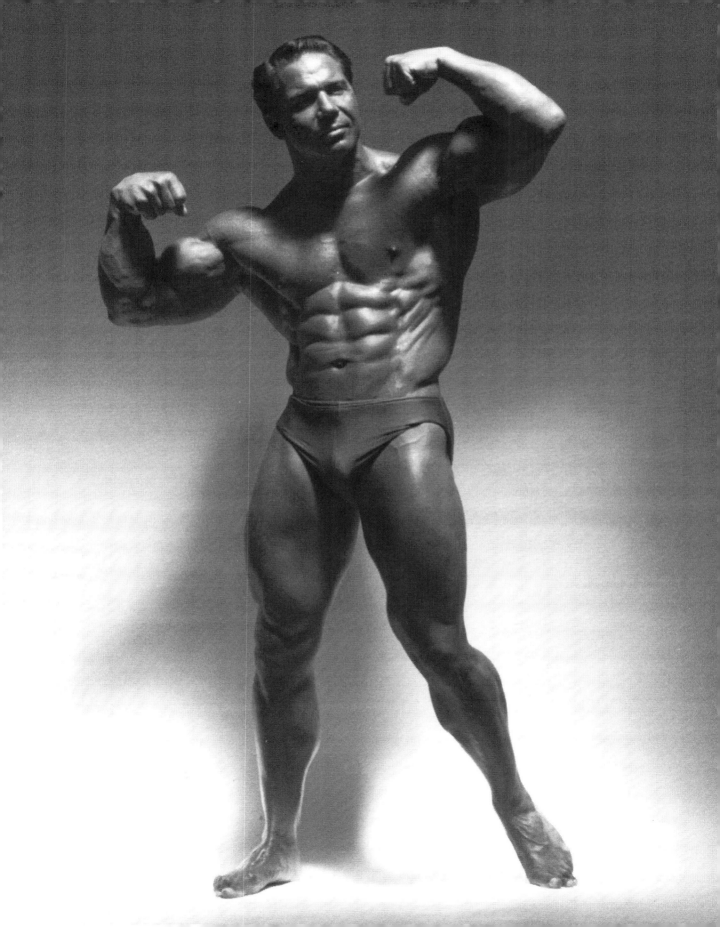

Image Number Forty-Two
Photographer - Leo Stern
At Stern's Gym, San Diego, CA
Circa 1970 thru 1971

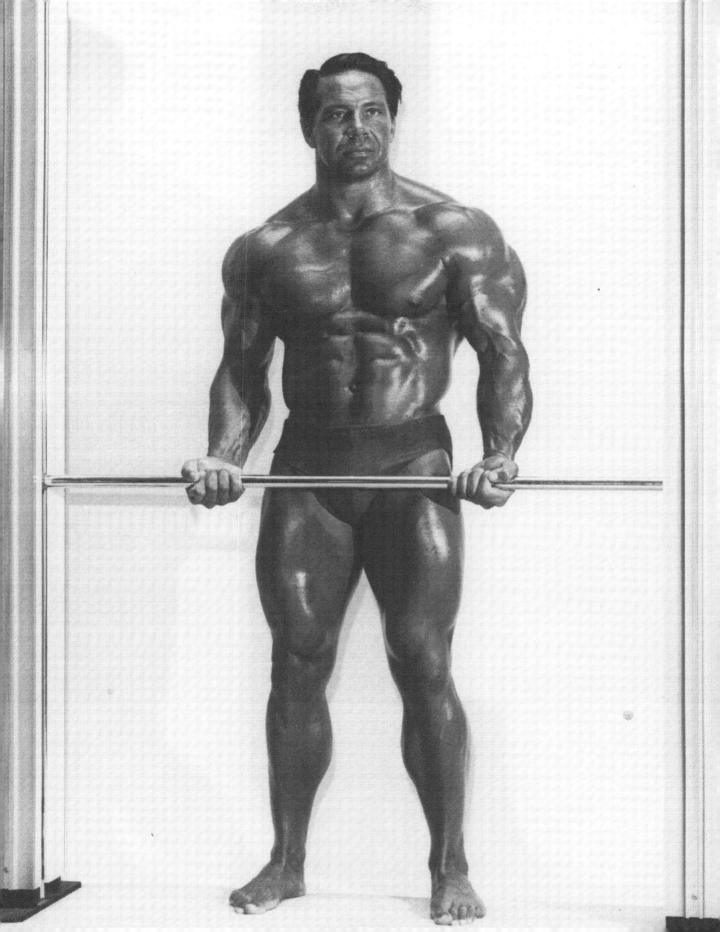

Image Number Forty-Three
Photographer - Leo Stern
At Stern's Gym, San Diego, CA
Circa 1970 thru 1971

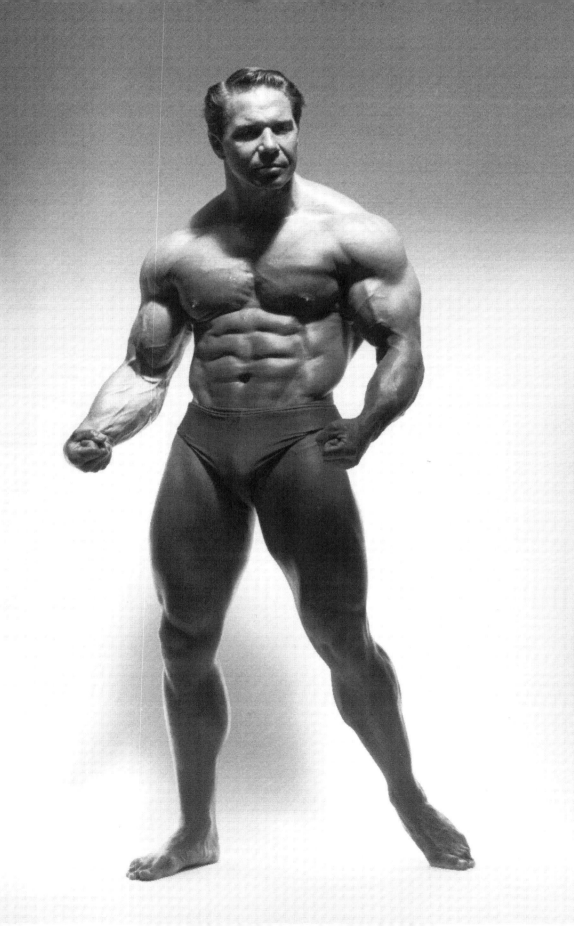

Image Number Forty-Four
Photographer - Leo Stern
At Stern's Gym, San Diego, CA
Circa 1970 thru 1971

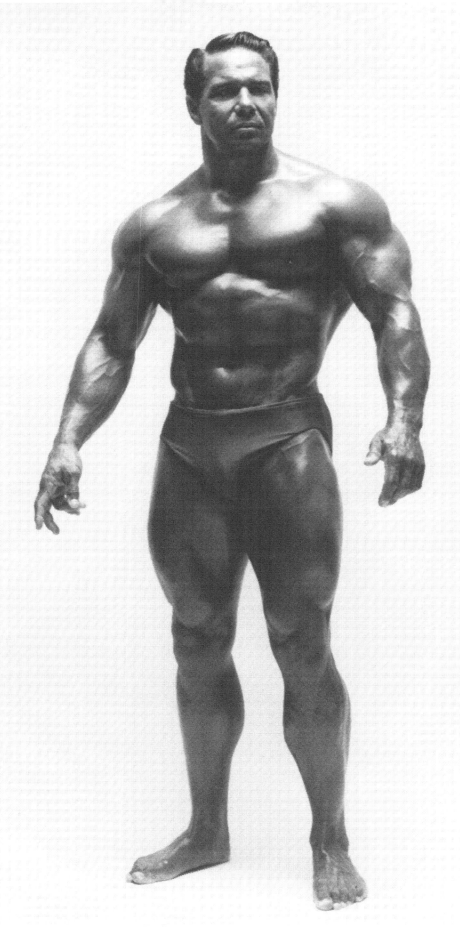

Image Number Forty-Five
Photographer - Leo Stern
At Stern's Gym, San Diego, CA
Circa 1970 thru 1971

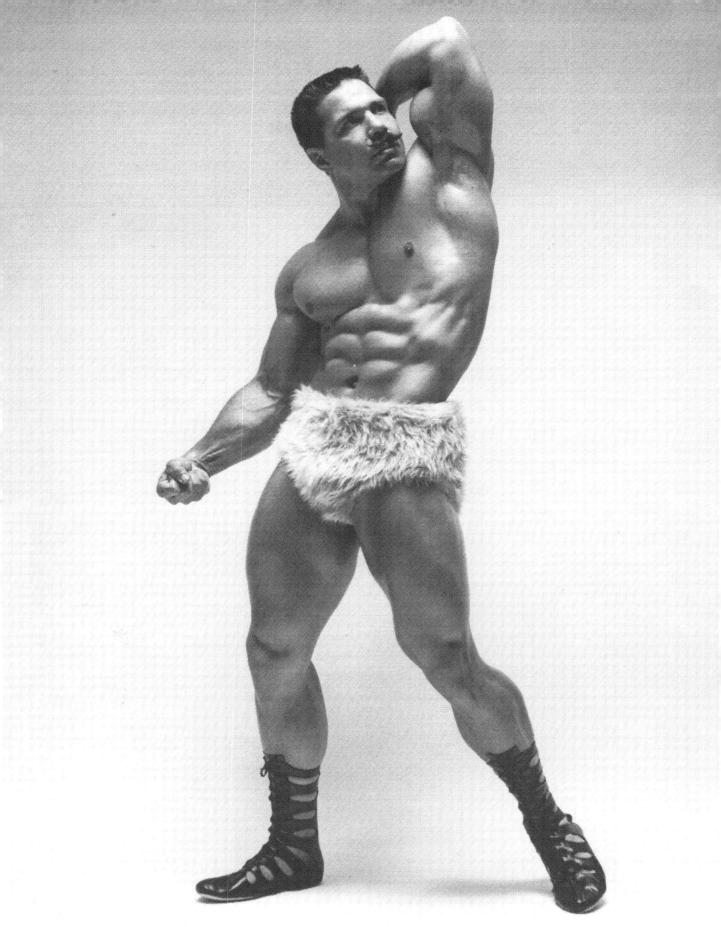

Image Number Forty-Six
Photographer - Leo Stern
At Stern's Gym, San Diego, CA
Circa 1963 thru 1966

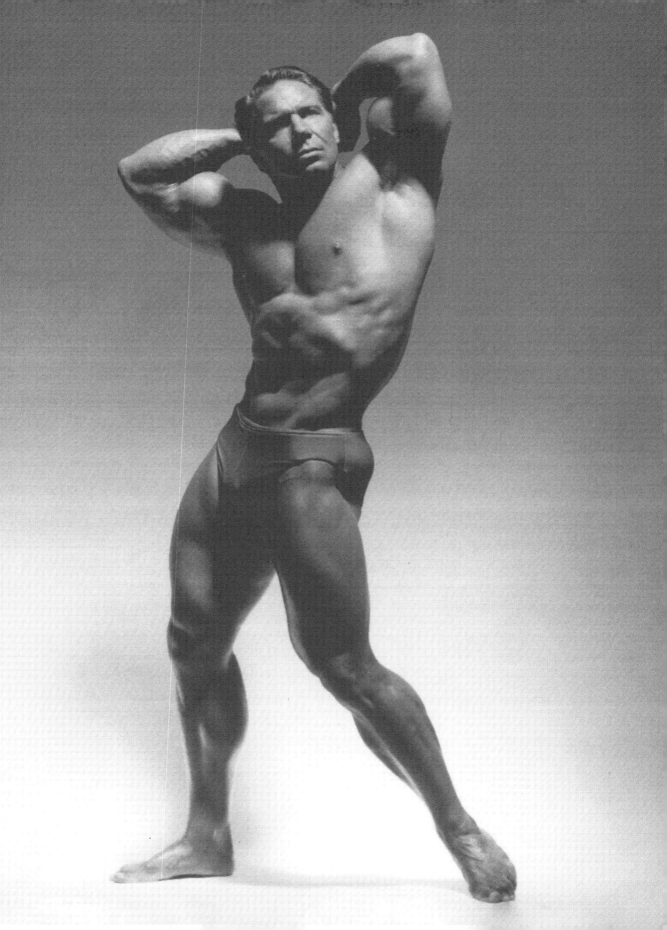

Image Number Forty-Seven
Photographer - Leo Stern
At Stern's Gym, San Diego, CA
Circa 1970 thru 1971

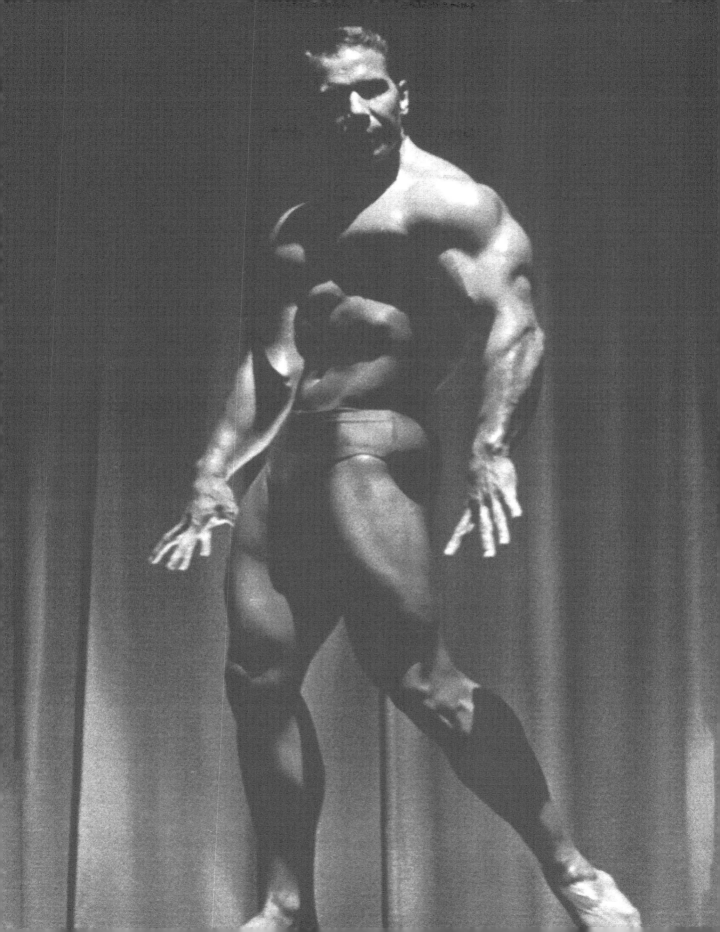

Image Number Forty-Eight
Photographer - George Coates
At the Embassy Auditorium, Los Angeles, CA
April 1971

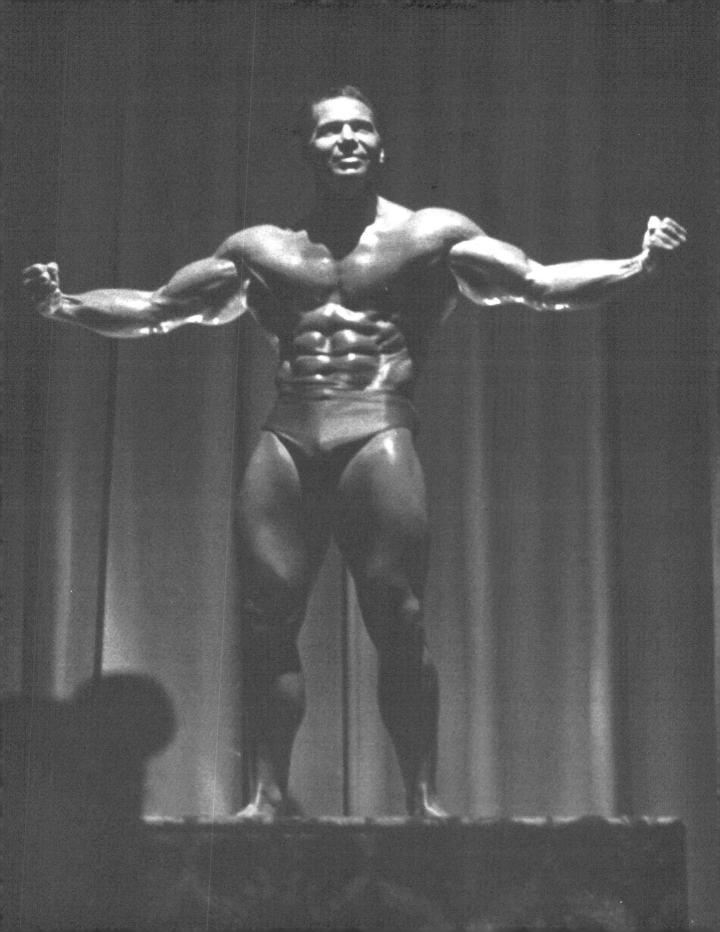

Image Number Forty-Nine
Photographer - George Coates
At the Embassy Auditorium, Los Angeles, CA
April 1971

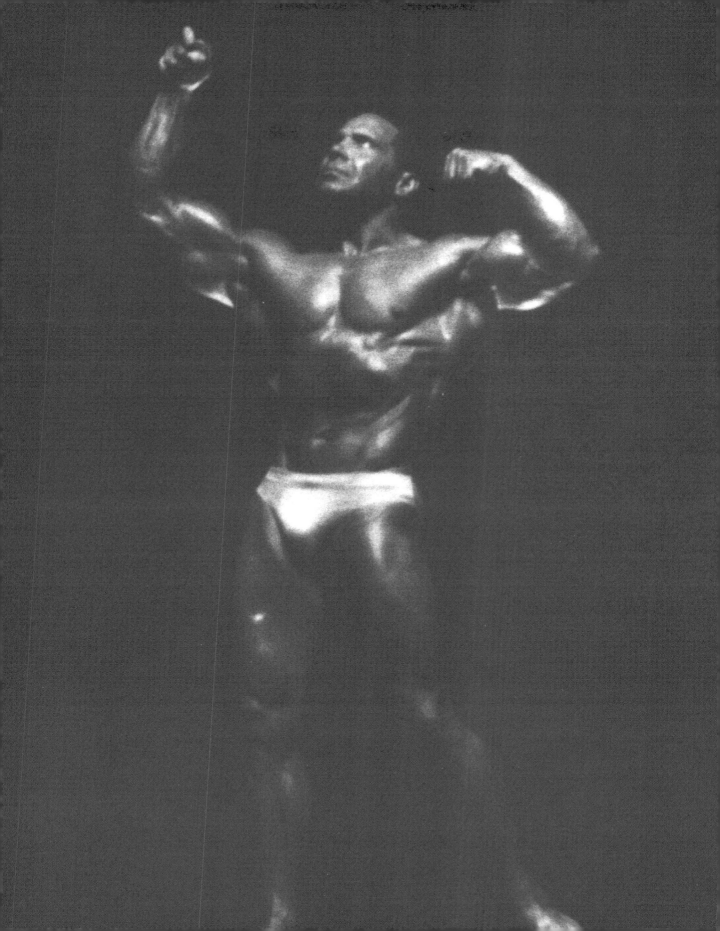

Image Number Fifty
Photographer - George Coates
At the Embassy Auditorium, Los Angeles, CA
April 1971

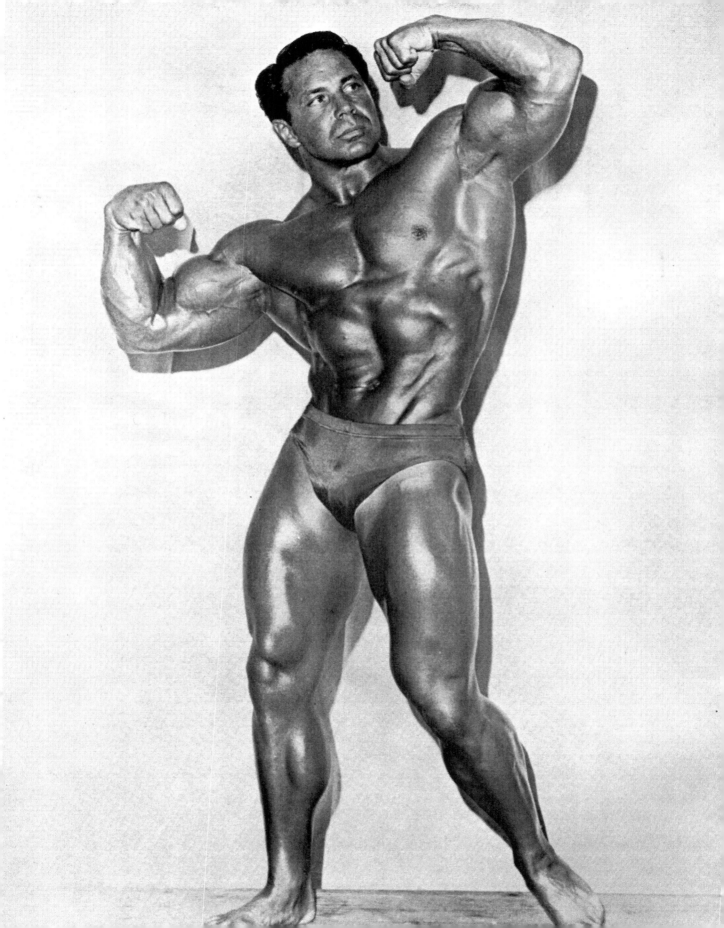

Image Number Fifty-One
Photographer - George Greenwood
At the 1971 NABBA Mr Universe Contest at
the Victoria Palace Theatre, London England

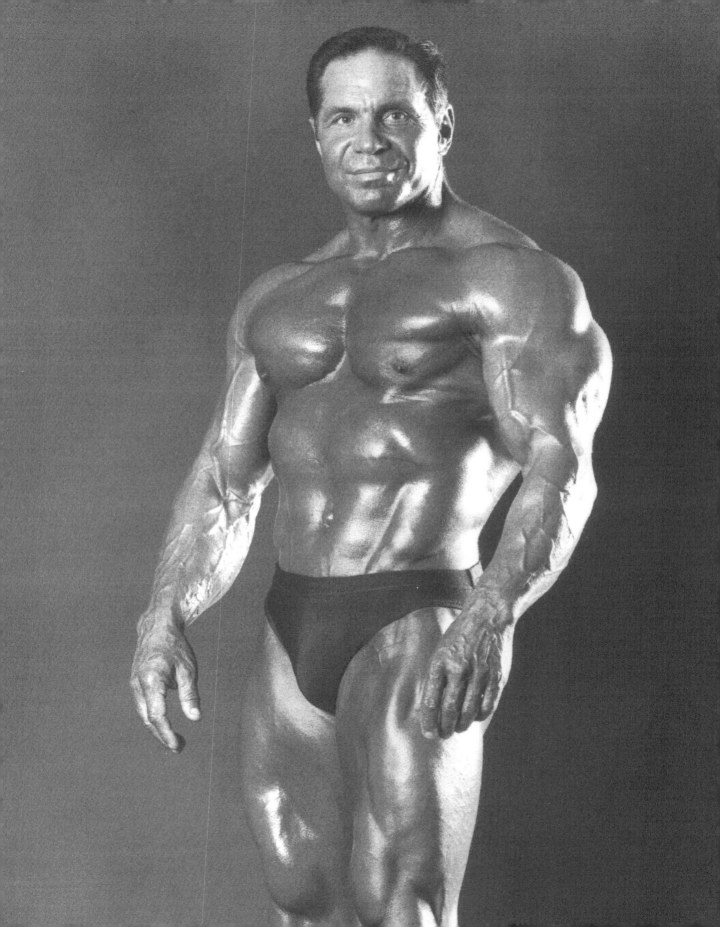

Image Number Fifty-Two
Photographer - Chris Lund
At John McGinnis' "Derby Classic" in Derby, England
As guest poser September 1987

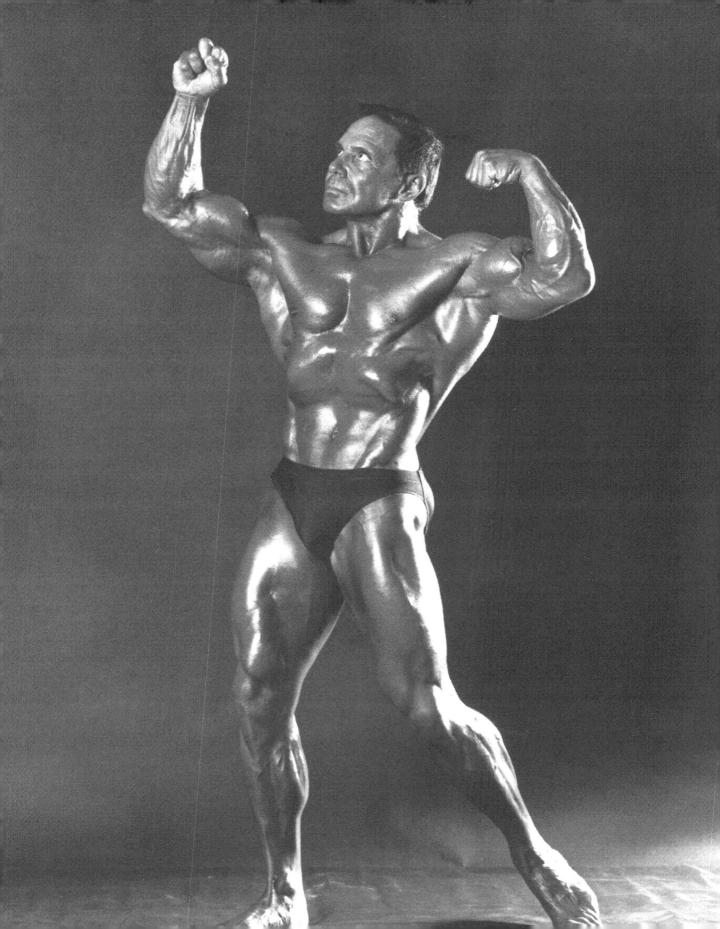

Image Number Fifty-Three
Photographer - Chris Lund
At John McGinnis' "Derby Classic" in Derby, England
As guest poser September 1987

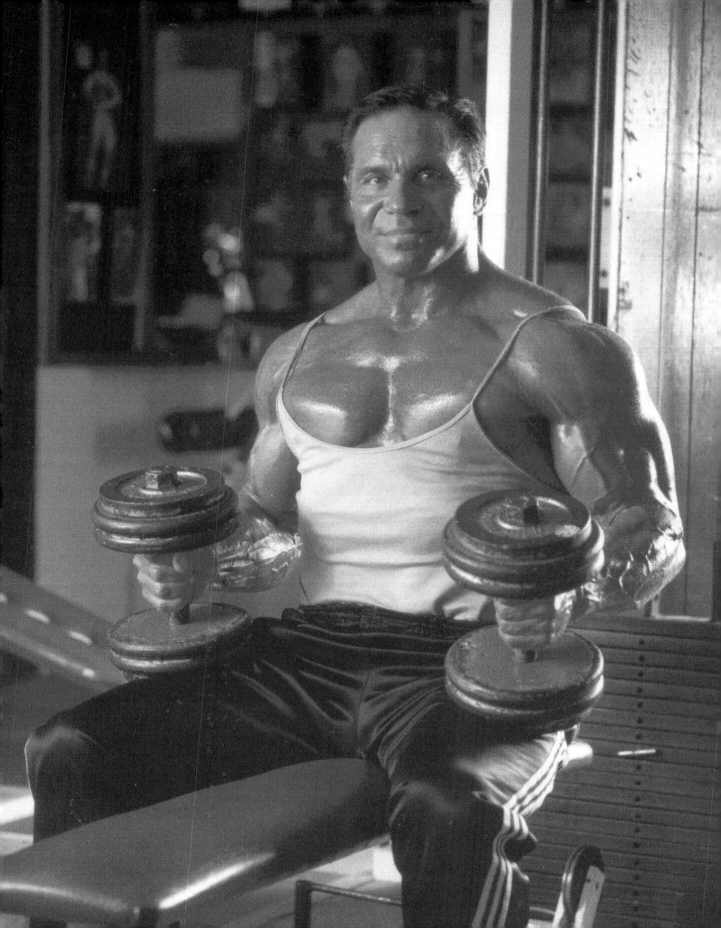

Image Number Fifty-Four
Photographer - Chris Lund
Seminar at John McGinnis' Gym in Derby, England at age 57!
September 1987

83586479R00062

Made in the USA
San Bernardino, CA
27 July 2018